A CAREGIVER'S GUIDE FOR ALZHEIMER'S

STAYING CONNECTED THROUGH ACTIVITIES

200 STAGE APPROPRIATE ACTIVITIES

IN HIS NAME

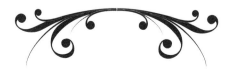

"

DO NOT ASK ME TO REMEMBER.
DON'T TRY TO MAKE ME UNDERSTAND.
LET ME REST AND KNOW YOU'RE WITH ME.
KISS MY CHEEK AND HOLD MY HAND.

I'M CONFUSED BEYOND YOUR CONCEPT.
I AM SAD AND SICK AND LOST.
ALL I KNOW IS THAT I NEED YOU
TO BE WITH ME AT ALL COST.

DO NOT LOSE YOUR PATIENCE WITH ME.
DO NOT SCOLD OR CURSE OR CRY.
I CAN'T HELP THE WAY I'M ACTING,
CAN'T BE DIFFERENT THOUGH I TRY.

JUST REMEMBER THAT I NEED YOU,
THAT THE BEST OF ME IS GONE.
PLEASE DON'T FAIL TO STAND BESIDE ME,
LOVE ME 'TIL MY LIFE IS GONE.

AUTHOR UNKNOWN

"

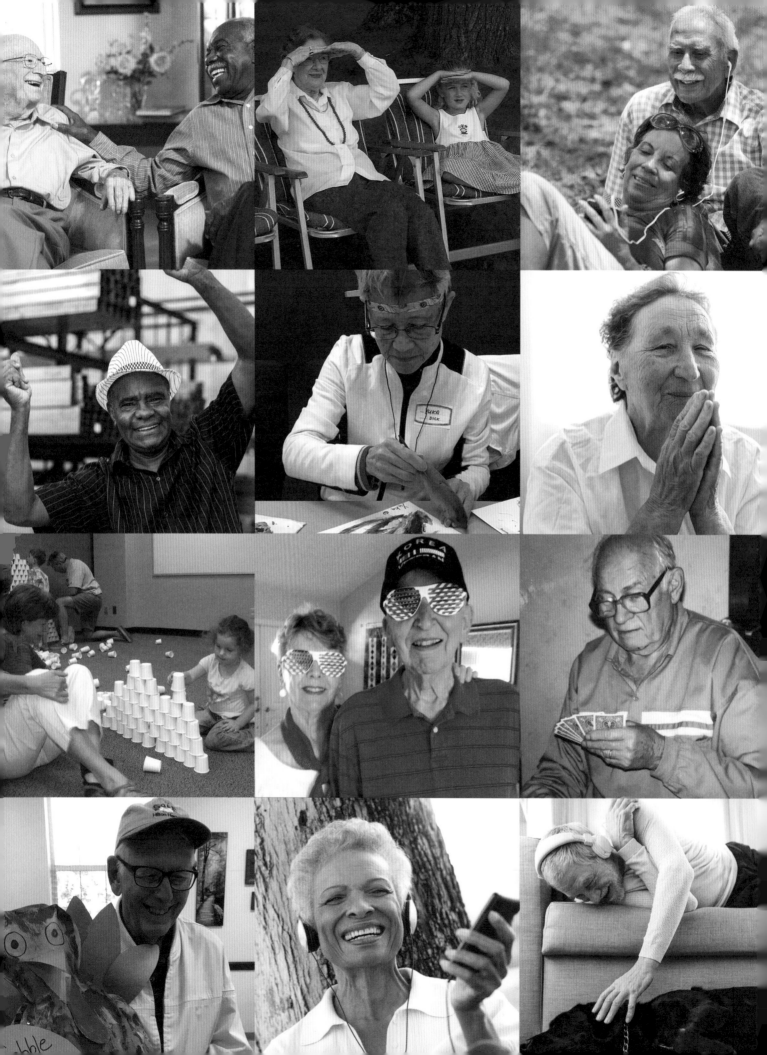

TABLE OF CONTENTS

TABLE OF CONTENTS

TABLE OF CONTENTS

TABLE OF CONTENTS

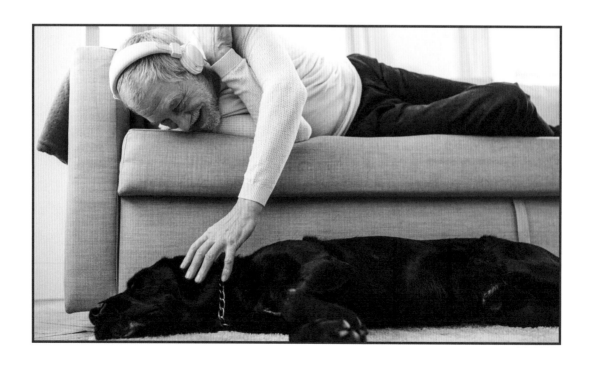

This Book Is Dedicated To
LUCILLE JESAITIS

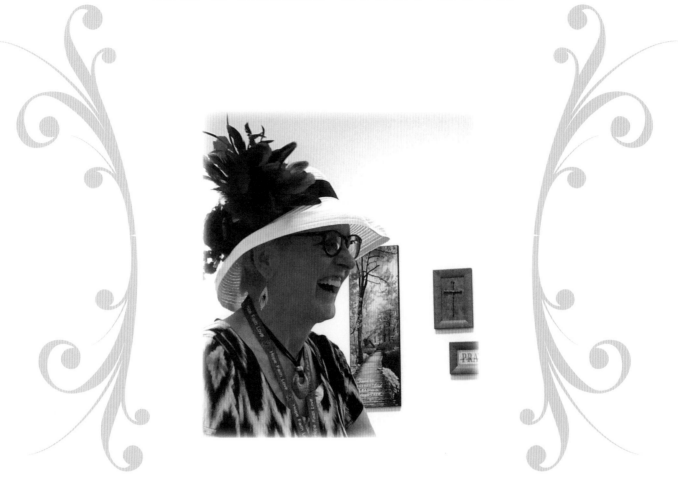

She was one of God's Shepherds, an example of God's Love to all of us.
She showed us even through suffering, God's presence abounded.
Lucille Jesaitis loved sharing her faith, adventure stories, unusual holiday
celebrations and her love of purple and crazy socks!! She had an
undying commitment to working with people with Alzheimer's.

Thank you Lucille for being the "heart and inspiration" for this book.

Lucille Jesaitis, June 29, 1942 – January 19, 2018

"Pray the hardest when it's hardest to pray"

INTRODUCTION AND ACKNOWLEDGEMENTS

By LINWOOD GALEUCIA

The true author of this book is <u>IN HIS NAME</u>. For as it is for all things, it is through The Lord, by Him and with Him that all things are created.

At a young age, I became aware that Jesus worked through others and me to serve those in need. Jesus often redirects life toward events of His will, not our will and for which we have little or no background, knowledge, experience, resources or sufficient ability to resolve.

The resolutions are always by The Lord providing the combination of individuals and resources needed to accomplish that which no individual alone possibly could.

This book is a perfect example. Each person who contributed in some manner to the content and activities within this book came from a different place with vastly different backgrounds and experiences.

In total we spent decades coping, treating and dealing with Alzheimer's Disease and Dementia. Each person traveled along a different path, one not of our choice, one we did not want, drawn together by a common thread.

Caregivers and Loved Ones who were forced into a battle against this common enemy, to band together, to work together, to serve the needs of each other, as we alone were unable to serve our needs.

Out of this experience came this book, some contributed knowingly, some unknowingly. All were guided by the hand, warmth and care of The Lord.

The Lord called upon numerous people to assist in the creation of this book. THEY INCLUDE:

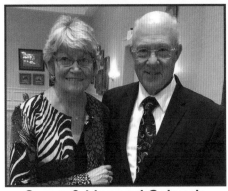
Susan & Linwood Galeucia
Teacher/Hospital Administrator

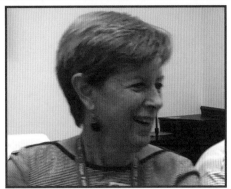
Jan Pandy
Teacher/Social Worker

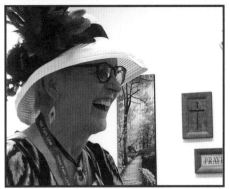
Lucille Jesaitis
Nurse

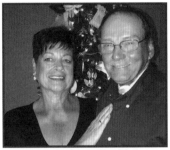
Vicki & Charlie Yates
Facilities Administrator/Teacher

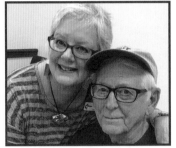
Kristie & Jim Faison
Activities Director/
Equipment Repair

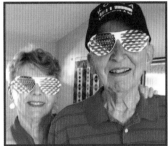
Jean & Chuck Hudson
Former Business Owners

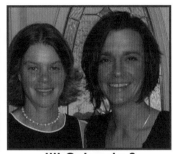
**Jill Galeucia &
Tina Underwood**
Bench Jeweler/
Education Administrator

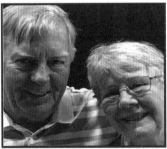
John & Betty Suprenant
Restaurant Owner/
Teacher

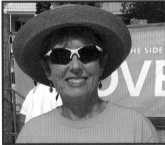
LaRae Donnellan
Communication Specialist

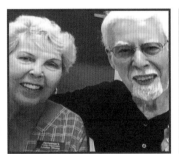
Louise & Carl Shuey
Executive Director Alzheimer's
Association/Airplane Mechanic

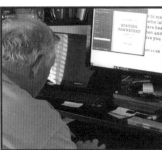
Bill Osborn
Electrical Engineer

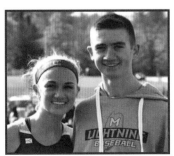
Hannah & Nick
Students

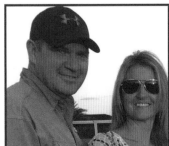
Mike & Angie Galeucia
Marketing Specialist/
Business Owner

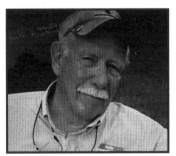
Peter Toppen
Paper Product Sales

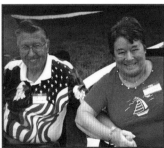
Jim & Penny Hoppe
Workman Comp. Manager/
Cosmetologist

Everyone you meet has an effect on your life

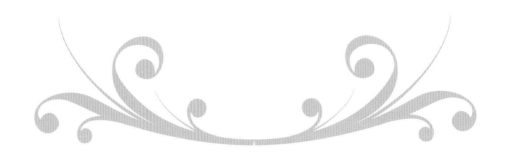

GOD IS PRESENT IN THE SIMPLE ACTS OF GIVING AND RECEIVING LOVE

Kenneth L. Carder

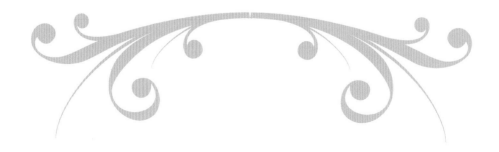

ACTIVITY GUIDELINES

- All activities are designed for the caregiver and the Loved One to do together as a combined activity and joint process.

- Activities are always directed toward getting a positive outcome for the Loved One and the caregiver.

- At all times be safe – be careful.
  Safety is paramount for:
    - The Loved One
    - The caregiver
    - All others concerned
  Do not take any risks of injury. Always consider the Loved One's limitations.

- This book is formatted to be an easy to follow, step by step instructional manual.
  Each activity includes:
    - Referring to care-receivers as the Loved One.
    - Supplies required.
    - An indication of stage appropriateness for the activity.
    - Step by step instructions.

- The "stage appropriateness" is only a general guideline and varies by individual. Sometimes the Loved One may not be interested in the activity and the caregiver can move on to another activity. Sometimes the caregiver will need to modify the activity to insure the Loved One experiences a positive outcome.

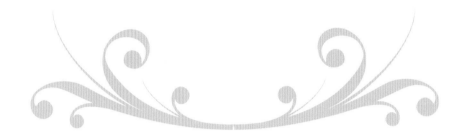

**Hope is not about believing
you can change things.
Hope is about believing you can
make a difference.**

Václav Havel

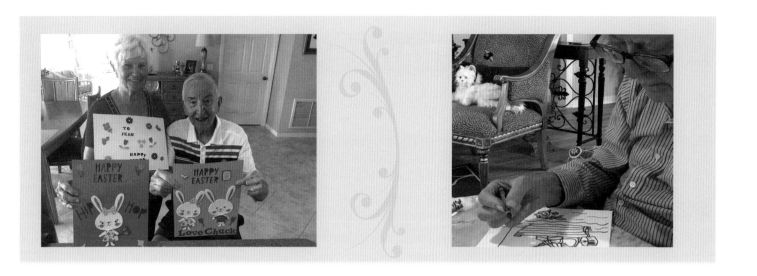

Creative *Is As*
Creative **D**oes

NO PRIOR ART EXPERIENCE NEEDED
"ART IS IN THE EYE OF THE BEHOLDER"
ART IS FOR ART'S SAKE AND IS TO BE ENJOYED

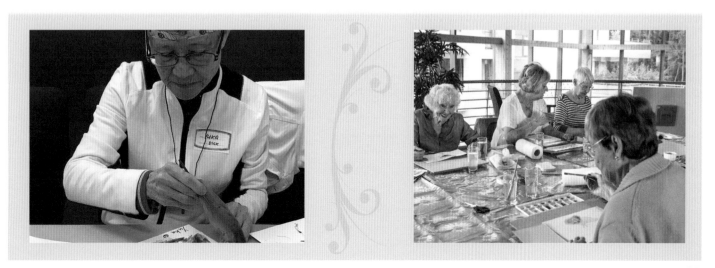

PLAYDOUGH AND STRAWS

A Fun, Colorful Activity

This activity will help with eye-hand coordination, fine motor skills and is a lot of fun!

SAFETY PRECAUTION!

✓ As the Loved One will be utilizing a variety of materials and small items, never leave the Loved One alone during this activity. It is a Loved One, caregiver participation activity.

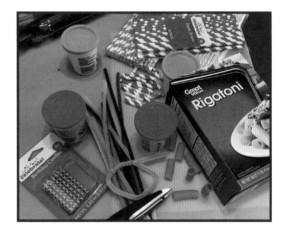

SUPPLIES:

- Plastic table cloth to protect the work surface
- Colorful straws
- Uncooked pasta, Ziti or Rigatoni
- Playdough the size of 2 or 3 softballs
- Small colorful cake candles
- Decorated, colorful, pipe cleaners
- Blunt nosed scissors (child scissors)

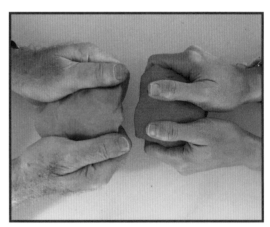

DIRECTIONS:

- Place the table cloth on the flat work surface.
- Remove the Playdough from their containers.
- Squish the Playdough into one (1) or two (2) piles, the size of a softball.
- Slightly flatten the Playdough pile.
- Take out the straws the caregiver has already cut into various lengths.
- Place pipe cleaners into Playdough any which way.
- Place straw pieces over the pipe cleaners.
- Take Ziti or Rigatoni out of box.
- Place anywhere in the Playdough.

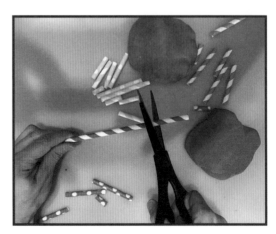

Playdough and Straws 2

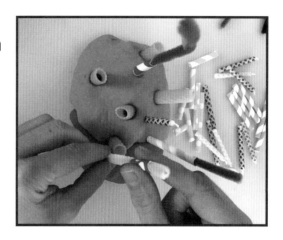

- Press uncooked pasta (like a stamp) into the Playdough to make impressions and designs.

- Try all kinds of things, like looping pipe cleaners from one piece of pasta to another or printing out your name with straws.

- Take pictures of you, the Loved One and your Playdough project to show family and friends.

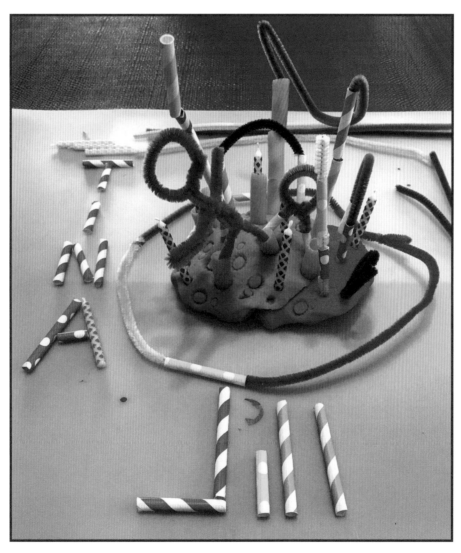

NOTE TO CAREGIVER:

- Take care to insure that the Loved One does not try to eat the Playdough. While the Playdough is non-toxic, non- irritating and non-allergenic, it tastes gross.

HOMEMADE PLAYDOUGH

Everyone enjoys playing with Playdough! It's soothing, feels good to the touch, is a great fine motor skill activity and a fun together activity. It's a good time to just sit, play and talk!
This is a non- toxic recipe for homemade Playdough or just buy it ready made.

SAFETY PRECAUTION!

✓ This recipe is non-toxic, but will require heating the ingredients on the stove.
  Be sure to supervise the Loved One if he/she is stirring on the stove.

SUPPLIES:

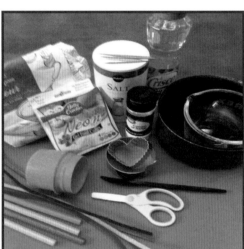

- Recipe
  - 1 cup flour
  - 1 tablespoon oil
  - 1/2 cup salt
  - 2 tsp. cream of tartar
  - Food coloring
  - 1 cup water
- Bowl/spoon/pan
- Wax paper
- Plastic container
- Straws, pipe cleaners
- Blunt scissors

DIRECTIONS:

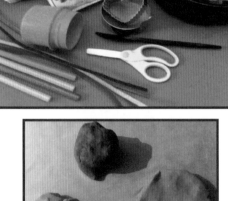

- Mix ingredients together.
- Stir over low heat until thick consistency.
- Take off heat and knead until cool.
  (It will be hot at first but will cool quickly)
- Play and enjoy.
- Store in air tight container or bag.
- DO NOT REFRIGERATE

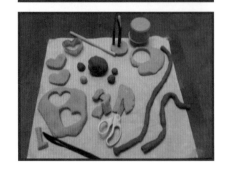

NOTE TO CAREGIVER:

- You can cut straws and/or pipe cleaners and stick in the Playdough. You can make letters, shapes and animals. A very good finger exercise is to cut the Playdough with children's blunt scissors. If you play with it… the Loved One will probably do the same!!!

HAPPY FACES

There are many approaches to this project. You can simply make a smiling face on paper or use several different materials.

SUPPLIES:

- Magic Markers
- Crayons
- Stickers
- Acrylic Paint
- Any round object to trace
- Paper
- Card Stock
- Yellow Paper Plates
- Paint Brush
- Yellow Highlighter
- Pencil

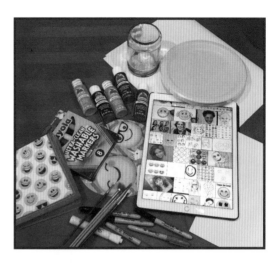

DIRECTIONS:

- Look for examples of happy faces. Happy faces are everywhere!!!

- Look in magazines, newspapers and other printed materials.

- Look for stickers.

- Search online using the computer and copy them for your personal use.

  - Option
    Make a face on a yellow paper plate with a magic marker or acrylic paint.

  - Option
    Trace a round object on card stock or white paper with a marker. Pencil in a face. Use a yellow highlighter to color the entire face. Then go over the pencil marks using a dark marker.

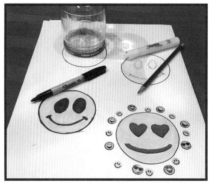

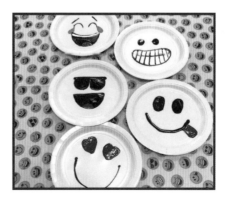

NOTE TO CAREGIVER:

- If the Loved One is not able to trace or color, try using stickers. Peel off the back of the sticker, and if necessary put it in place and have the Loved One "tap, tap, tap" with their finger to make it stick.

PAINT CHIPS

Caregivers can pick up a large variety of paint chip samples, free at paint stores and paint departments in large box stores such as Walmart, Lowes, etc. There are many different ways that paint chips can be used. Some are noted in this "paint chip" activity.

SAFETY PRECAUTION!

✓ When using scissors (preferably blunt nosed), magic markers and glue always supervise the Loved One.

SUPPLIES:

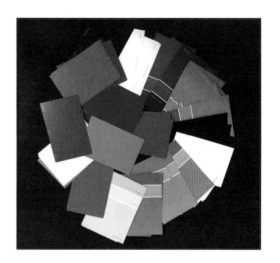

• Pick out an assortment of paint chip samples. Once you choose a color pick two (2) of the same color and shade and then pick out two (2) of an entirely different color and so on. Do not pick out a similar color or shade of the same color.

• Stickers

• Various colored magic markers

• Glue stick

• White or colored paper/ card stock

• Blunt nosed scissors

DIRECTIONS:
ACTIVITY NO. 1 BOOKMARKS

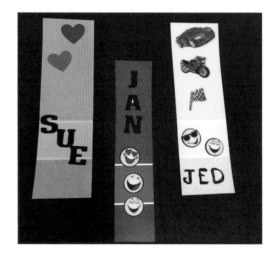

• Make bookmarks by cutting paint chips to size and decorating with stickers.

DIRECTIONS: ACTIVITY NO. 2 MATCHING GAME

- Play a matching game to match paint chips of the same distinctive color.

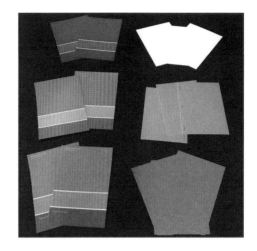

DIRECTIONS: ACTIVITY NO. 3 PUZZLE

- Use two or more paint chips, line them up, draw a picture or design across them. Separate the chips and have the Loved One line them up like a puzzle.

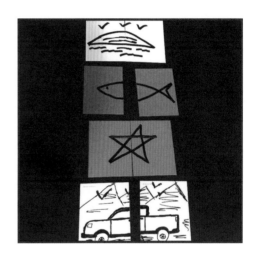

DIRECTIONS: ACTIVITY NO. 4 DESIGNS

- Cut the paint chips into different sizes and shapes. Glue them onto a piece of paper to make a design.

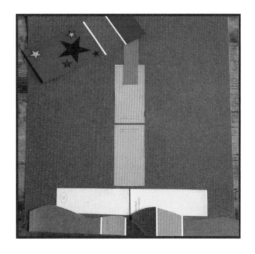

NOTE TO CAREGIVER:

- Activities using paint chips can be very simple or more complex depending on the skill level of the Loved One. Start with a simple activity. Remember you want the Loved One to feel successful and enjoy the activity. The Loved One may create their own use for the paint chips.

ALCOHOL INK STAMPING

Decorating Tiles

This easy art project produces great results at a low cost. No one can make a mistake. Only lots of fun!

SAFETY PRECAUTION!

✓ Keep and store Alcohol Ink safely from the Loved One. When using, supervise the Loved One at all times. Do not permit the Loved One to spray the hair spray or lacquer spray on the final art piece.

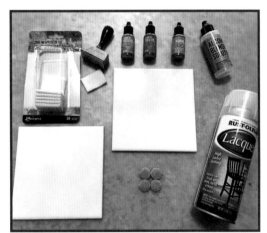

SUPPLIES:

(Available at craft store)

• Cost: $10-$15

• Variety of alcohol ink colors (3 are enough to start)

• Alcohol-blending solution or rubbing alcohol

• Ink stamper and pads made for alcohol-ink use

• Square white tiles (4 ¼ inch or 6 inch)

• Small felt pads with sticky backing to use as feet

• Clear lacquer spray (or hairspray)

• Plastic mat to protect work surface

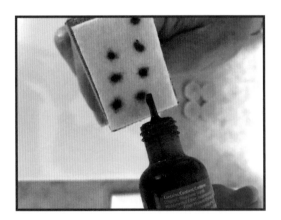

DIRECTIONS:
OPTION NO. 1 INK DROP

• Clean the top surface of a tile with alcohol and paper towel.

• Place a white ink pad on the ink stamper.

• Apply 12-18 drops of one color ink on the pad surface, leaving space between drops.

• Dab the stamped pad on the white tile, leaving spaces. Allow ink to dry 20-30 seconds.

• Replace the ink pad with a clean one, and apply another color.

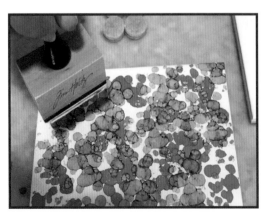

DIRECTIONS:
OPTION NO. 2 INK FLOW

- Take a new tile and clean the surface, as before.

- Place a large drop (or several small drops) of ink directly on the tile.

- Then try one or more of these methods:
  - Tip the tile so the ink flows in different directions.
  - Blow the ink across the tile with a straw.
  - Spread the ink with a feather.
  - Use a toothpick or hard end of a paintbrush to run a line of ink across the tile.

- Let the ink dry before applying a different color.

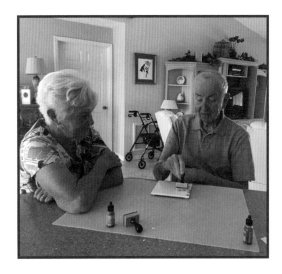

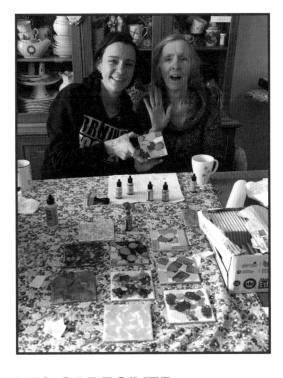

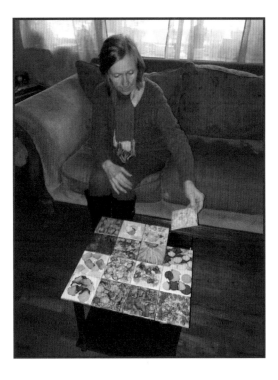

NOTE TO CAREGIVER:

- If the ink drops onto something that shouldn't be inked, then use the alcohol solution and a paper towel to clean it up.

- Do not wash the tiles unless you already finished them with a few coats of lacquer. Please apply lacquer in a well ventilated area or outside. You can apply these same procedures to other shaped tiles or nonporous materials, such as glossy paper, glass, metal or ceramic. When the tiles are done you can add felt pads to the back of the tiles.

COLORING/PAINTING

"Artistic talent not required"

There are numerous activities and methods to color and paint. Included in this write up are only a few. All activities with thought and practice can be modified to the needs and capabilities of the Loved One.

SAFETY PRECAUTION!

✓ Take care that all coloring and painting products are non – toxic. Water based, washable paints are preferred. Keep open paint containers covered & secured when not in use. Supervise the Loved One at all times.

SUPPLIES:

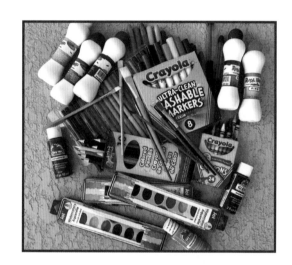

- Include but not limited to:
  - Paper, tracing paper, cardboard & card stock
  - Water colors, finger paint & acrylic paint
  - Crayons, magic markers, colored pencils, colored bingo daubers
  - Paint brushes, Q-tips
  - Coloring books, clip art & computer applications
  - iPad, tablets

DIRECTIONS:
ACTIVITY NO. 1 COLORING

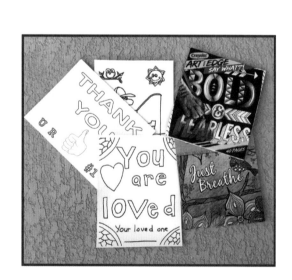

- Select topics that are enjoyable for the Loved One.
- Select pictures that are not too complex or detailed.
- Select coloring books that are not childish.
- If you cannot locate a suitable coloring book, try clip art in the following manner:
  - On a computer search for free clip art.
  - Select a picture and click on it.
  - Print out the picture.
  - If that does not work then use tracing paper and trace the picture. **(Do not break copyright laws in use of this material).**

• Color with supplies of your choice. The Loved One's ability to color or hold an implement may be affected, or reduced by a number of factors. So modify, modify & modify.
Some suggestions:

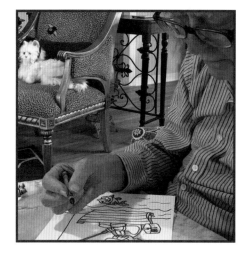

  - Coloring "inside the lines" is not essential.

  - Assist the Loved One slightly.

  - Reduce the number of choices confronting the Loved One by handing them one color at a time.

  - You do a small part then they do a part.

  - If that does not work see coloring modified Activity 2.

DIRECTIONS: ACTIVITY NO. 2 MODIFIED COLORING WITH DAUBERS

• First make a simple line drawing.

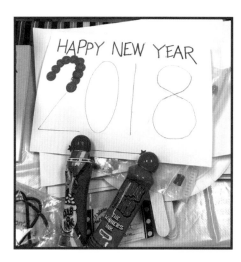

• Utilize Bingo Daubers. Daubers are easier to hold.
Daubers technically do not do coloring but can be "daubed".

• Select a Dauber and press it once on any line of the line drawing and repeat. (It is ok if the Loved One misses the line).

DIRECTIONS: ACTIVITY NO. 3 PAINTING

• Select painting projects that are enjoyable.
Options include:

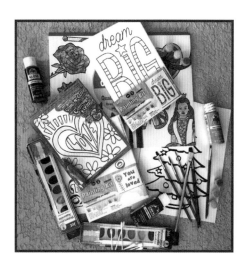

  - Paint kits. Kits are available in dollar type stores, big box stores such as Walmart, craft stores and on-line.

  - Paint books.

  - Make your own drawings to paint, utilizing free clip art (described in the coloring activity) on card stock.

NOTE TO CAREGIVER:

• There is a fine line between assisting and doing a project "for" the Loved One.

• One modification to try when painting is to substitute the use of Q-tips in place of paint brushes.
Q-tips are easier to hold and easier to paint with. Another thought is to use washable finger paints.

STENCILING

This is an easy art form that gets very good results.

SUPPLIES:

- Stencils
- Stencil brush
- Bingo dauber
- Sponge roller
- Colored pencils, pens or felt marker
- Washable acrylic craft paints
- Stencil tape
- Card stock or paper
- Plastic protective covering for table if needed

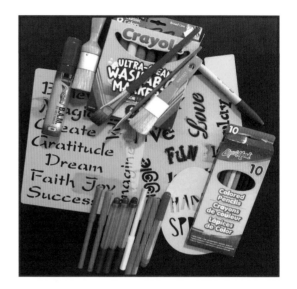

DIRECTIONS:

- Select stencil.
- Tape it to paper or card stock.
- Select sponge roller or dauber.
- Apply paint to stencil.
- Or select pencil, pen or marker.
- Color in open area of stencil.
- You can just make art or create cards or signs.

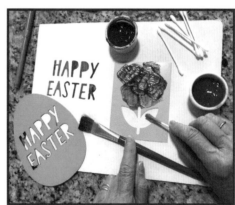

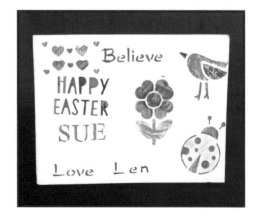

NOTE TO CAREGIVER:

- Supplies are readily available at dollar type stores, box stores and arts and craft stores.

MILK AND FOOD COLOR ART

Easy, Fun & Easy To Clean Up

This activity is simple yet produces beautiful results. All items utilized most likely are found in your kitchen.

SUPPLIES:

- Milk
- Laundry Detergent
- Assorted Food Color
- Plastic Plate – Clear
- Small Plastic Bowl
- Q-tips

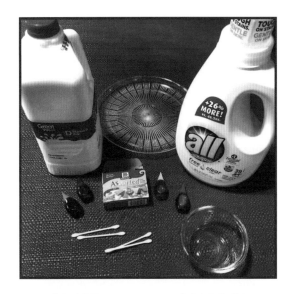

DIRECTIONS:

- Pour milk onto plastic plate.
- Place one or two drops of each food color on the milk.
- Pour a little detergent into a small bowl.
- Dip the Q-tip a little into the detergent.
- Touch the Q-tip with the detergent end on a color on the plate.
- Repeat for each color.
- Swirl the colors together.

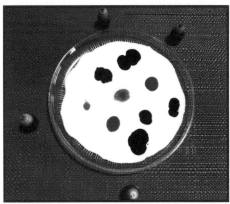

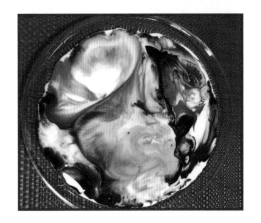

NOTE TO CAREGIVER:

- You can take pictures with your cellphone and you can pour out milk and start all over again.

PENCIL JAR

Practical, useful yet cute & fun

SAFETY PRECAUTION!

✓ If you choose to utilize small decorative objects such as beads, old jewelry or buttons be aware they may pose a choking hazard. Keep all small objects in a covered container and in a safe place.

SUPPLIES:

- Plastic jar (glass if safe to do so) about the size of a regular jelly jar.
- Yarn (multicolored or fancy textured yarn is nice)
- Tacky glue
- Small paper plate
- Scissors
- Craft paint brush
- Pencils
- Small decorative items such as beads, jewelry, buttons, fabric trim, etc. if desired.

DIRECTIONS:

- Pour about two (2) tablespoons of glue onto the paper plate.
- With the paint brush, brush the glue on the outside lower one quarter (¼)of the jar. Be sure to go all around the jar.
- Starting at the bottom of the jar wrap the yarn continually around the jar until you reach the top of where the glue was spread.

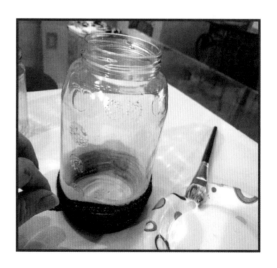

Pencil Jar 2

- With the paint brush apply glue to the next one quarter (¼) of the jar.

- Wrap the yarn around the jar as before.

- Continue this process until you reach the top of the jar.

- Trim off the yarn at the top.

- You may choose to continue to decorate the jar by glueing on small items such as beads, old jewelry, buttons or fabric trim.

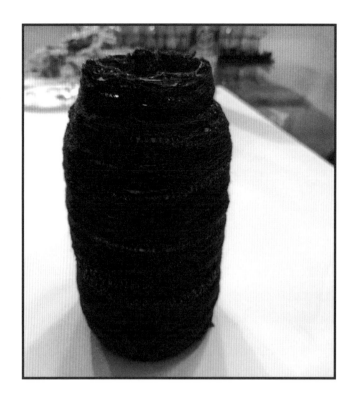

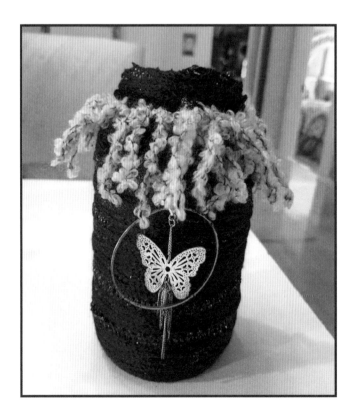

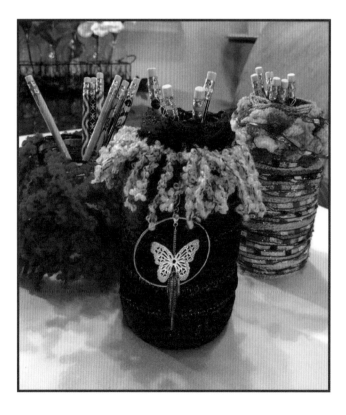

NOTE TO CAREGIVER:

- This size jar can now be utilized to hold the pencils (or pens). You can continue this activity by decorating all sizes of plastic containers for various storage needs.

PAINTING WITH FEATHERS

A new experience for most

You may be surprised at the many different ways each painting will vary whether one person does several different paintings or several different people each do one painting.

This type of painting does not require any art experience or ability. It is simply a fun easy project to do.

SUPPLIES:

- Plastic or paper table covering to protect the work surface
- Blank sheets of card stock or cardboard
- Washable, water soluble "finger" paint
- Package of feathers from craft store, Walmart, Target, etc.
- Paper plates
- Towel to clean up paint drops or spills
- Plastic spoon
- Paint stirrer

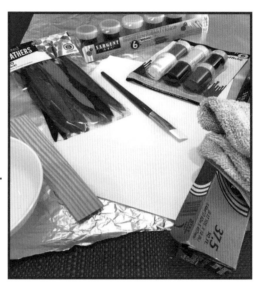

DIRECTIONS:

- The caregiver should prepare the paint by using the plastic spoon to scoop out each different color paint onto a paper plate.

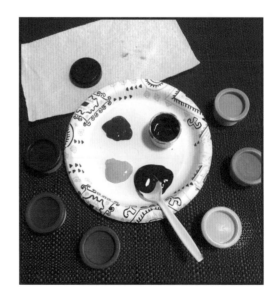

- Select one feather and give it to the Loved One.

- Show or have the Loved One dip just the tip of the feather into one of the paint colors.

- If the paint appears to be too thick, thin it with water.

- Have the Loved One dab, swirl and drag the paint feather any which way across a blank piece of paper.

- A new feather should be used if the Loved One wants to change from one color to another.

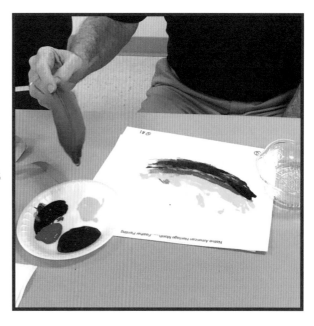

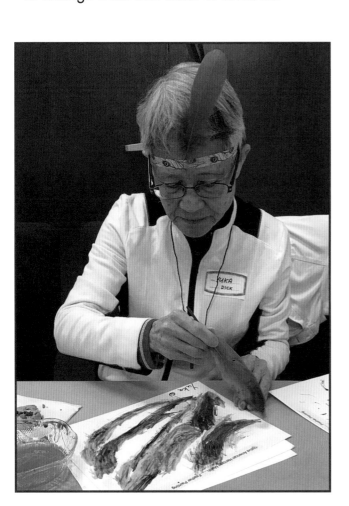

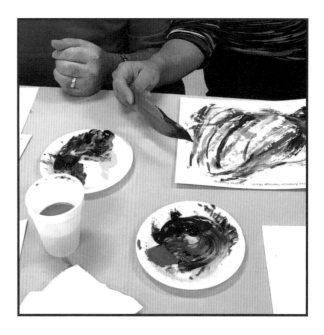

NOTE TO CAREGIVER:

- As with all art projects in this book, there is no wrong way, better way, or best way to do this project. If the Loved One cannot get the idea of how to start the activity you can take a feather and paint and the Loved One can then follow the lead of the caregiver.

- Also remember to take a picture of the painting with a cellphone or camera to send to others, or talk about with the Loved One at another time.

TAPE ART

This is an activity that may end up looking a little like a stained glass window.

SAFETY PRECAUTION!

✓ Prepare the work area and the Loved One for working with paints and the likelihood of spills.

SUPPLIES:

• Canvas board – about 8"x10" in size

• Scotch tape

• Acrylic jars of paint of different colors

• Paint brush

• Cup for water to clean brushes

• Plastic table cloth – something to protect the surface area

• Paper towels

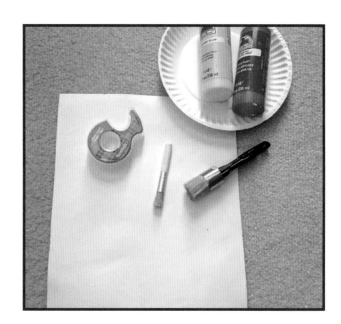

DIRECTIONS:

• Place the canvas board on a table with protective covering.

• Pull off a length of tape and work with the Loved One to place it in any direction from one side to the other.

• Pull off another length of tape and tape it in a different direction on the canvas. Do not be worried if it intersects or overlaps other tape, this can be beneficial.

• Repeat the process while leaving a number of different areas of the canvas exposed.

• Put a little bit of one color of paint into the paint jar lid.

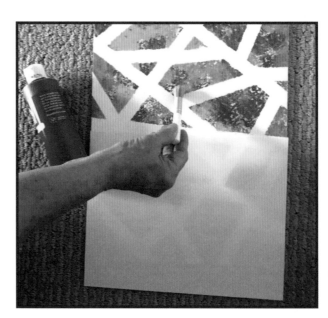

Tape Art 2

- Dip a paint brush into the paint and have the Loved One dab it on one or a few of the exposed canvas areas.

- Clean the brush with water and paper towel.

- Repeat the process in a different canvas area with a different color.

- Continue the process until all areas of the exposed canvas are covered.

- Let the paint dry completely.

- When dry, the Loved One can pull off each piece of tape and see the design.

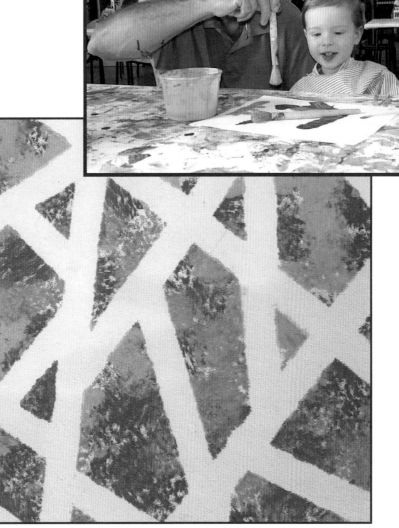

NOTE TO CAREGIVER:

- Do not be concerned when the Loved One is applying the paint if the tape also gets covered. It will not affect the results. Just let the Loved One dab the paint all over the canvas board.

ZEN TREASURE GARDEN

SAFETY PRECAUTION!

✓ Watch that the Loved One does not put any small objects in their mouth. Also the sand can be a choking hazard.

SUPPLIES:

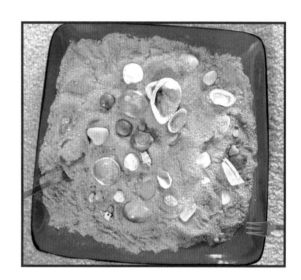

- Play sand (specifically sold for children is natural, non-toxic, will not dry out and comes in various colors)
- Plastic round shallow container, possibly with a lid
- Small plastic fork or tiny house plant rake
- Small smooth rocks
- Medium size glass flat marble vase fillers
- Coins and medals

DIRECTIONS:

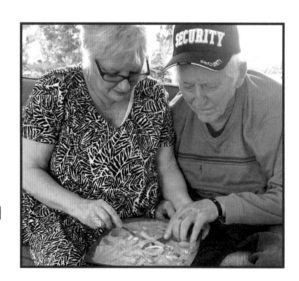

- Clean and sanitize, as possible, all items to be placed in the sand.
- Pour sand about 1 ½ to 2 inches deep into the container.
- Place the objects into the sand.
- Cover the objects – treasures with sand.
- The Loved One can now use the small fork or rake to find the treasures.
- You may want to remove each object as it is found and place it on the table.
- You can talk about what is found and count the objects.

PLASTIC JUG BALL CATCHER

Many people enjoy playing catch. Traditionally we play catch with a glove and ball. In this activity the Loved One and caregiver will create a jug ball catcher and play catch with a very soft lightweight ball or round object.

SAFETY PRECAUTION!

✓ When you make your jug ball catcher, cover all rough or sharp edges with duct tape. When playing catch, only throw a very soft, lightweight object so that if it hits someone it will absolutely not hurt. Hard, rigid or weighted items should never be used.

SUPPLIES:

- Two (2) one (1) gallon plastic jugs
- Scissors
- Duct tape
- Very soft balls or make paper balls
- Stickers

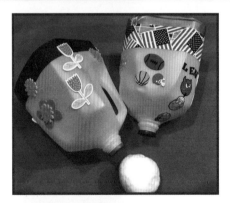

DIRECTIONS:

- Before you start with this activity, cut off the bottom of the jug and tape the sharp edge with duct tape.
- The Loved One can now decorate the two (2) jugs with duct tape and stickers.
- Toss the soft object to each other and catch with the jug-catcher.

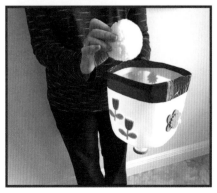

NOTE TO CAREGIVER:

- If the Loved One is a little unstable while standing, the Loved One and the caregiver can play catch while both are sitting down.

CLOTHES PINS

Clip-type clothes pins and assorted lids… that's all you need for a great fine motor skill activity. You can even turn it into a game for the Loved One.

SAFETY PRECAUTION!

✓ Do not use very small lids or other items that could result in choking.

SUPPLIES:

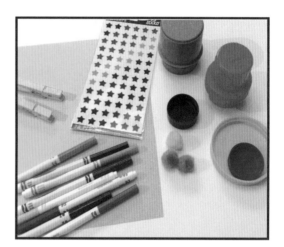

- Clip-type clothes pins (Dollar Tree, Walmart)
- Stickers
- Magic markers
- A collection of tops and lids from:
  - Gallon water/milk jugs
  - Peanut butter jars
  - Laundry soap containers
  - Salad dressing bottles
- Cotton balls and other lightweight items
- Container to store items

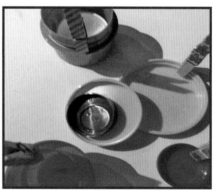

DIRECTIONS:

- Decorate the clothes pins with markers and/or stickers.
- Wash the lids and tops. Place them, the cotton balls and light items on the table.
- Use the clothes pins to pick up the items.
- Drop the items into a container after picking them up.

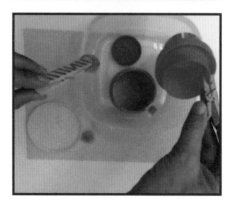

NOTE TO CAREGIVER:

- Can you think of other things to do with clothes pins?

I'LL DO ONE... THEN YOU DO ONE!

A magnetic popsicle stick matching game!

Stage Appropriate:
Early & Middle

Number of Participants:
1 to 1

This activity is easy, fun and as simple or difficult as you want for the Loved One. You will surely think of some different magnetic pieces to use to create a fun activity.

SAFETY PRECAUTION!

✓ Using small magnetic pieces can pose a choking hazard. Wooden pieces and popsicle sticks may look like food items. Do not leave the Loved One alone while making this activity.

SUPPLIES:

(Supplies can be found at Walmart/Dollar Tree)

- Large colored popsicle sticks/tongue depressors
- Magnetic strips with adhesive backing.
- Optional: other wooden shapes
- Cookie sheet
- Scissors

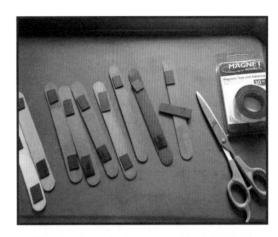

DIRECTIONS:

- Use an assortment of colored popsicle sticks.
- Stick magnetic pieces, strips or squares onto the backs of popsicle sticks.
- Stick them on a cookie sheet.
- Tell the Loved One that you will make a design and then below yours, he/she will copy it.

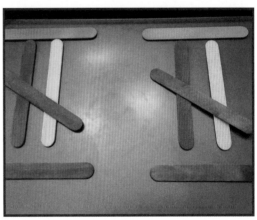

NOTE TO CAREGIVER:

- For a successful experience start with very simple designs and then increase the difficulty level if needed. Cookie sheets make this extra fun and easy for the Loved One to use and see the design.

RUBBER STAMPING

Rubber stamping is a method to transfer images, words, or letters from a pre-made rubber stamp onto many different items. This activity can be modified in many ways to keep the Loved One involved and gain a sense of accomplishment. When selecting stamps consider ones with phrases that assist the Loved One to communicate. Example: "Thank You" or "I Love You".

SAFETY PRECAUTION!

✓ If you utilize a pre-prepared solution to clean the rubber stamp or the work area, read and follow the precautions on the container. Utilize acid free, non-toxic dye ink pads only.

SUPPLIES:

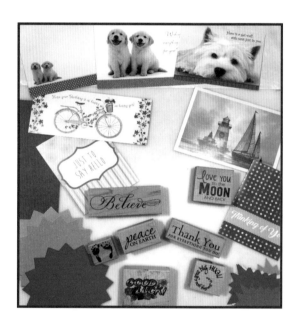

- Rubber stamp mounted on a block of wood
- Dye ink pad
- Copy paper, card stock and/ or greeting card
- Rubber gloves
- Mod Podge for finishing touches
- Plastic protector for the surface you will be working on

DIRECTIONS:

- Prepare a flat stable work area by covering it with a protector preferably plastic or a discardable table cloth.
- Take a piece of paper, card stock or greeting card and lay it out on the flat surface.
- Have the Loved One select a rubber stamp.
- Stamp the rubber stamp on to the dye-ink pad until the stamp is fully covered.
- The Loved One can stamp the inked rubber stamp where desired as often as desired.

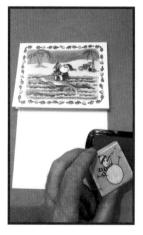
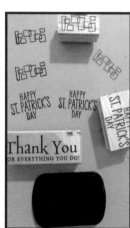

Rubber Stamping 2

• The Loved One can make cards, signs, messages or simply stamp, stamp, stamp. In later stages assistance can be provided at each step, even where to stamp, but if possible let them stamp, stamp, stamp.

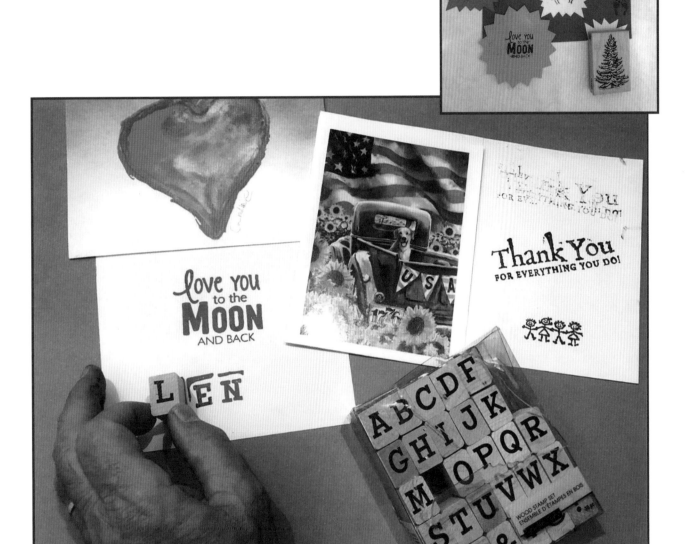

NOTE TO CAREGIVER:

• Rubber stamps can be expensive. If buying new, check on the prices in a variety of stores and online. Also search out used ones in thrift stores and consignment shops as well as yard and garage sales. Another option is to find a rubber stamping hobbyist and borrow or share rubber stamps.

DECORATING CLIPBOARDS

Clipboards are one of the most useful items you can imagine and such fun to personalize and make together. Using a clipboard to secure paper of any kind to the board, enables the Loved One to better manage tasks.

SAFETY PRECAUTION!

✓ Care should be taken relating to supplies that might go into the Loved One's mouth such as: paint, brushes, magic markers, glue stick, Mod Podge. Please do not leave the Loved One alone with these supplies.

SUPPLIES:

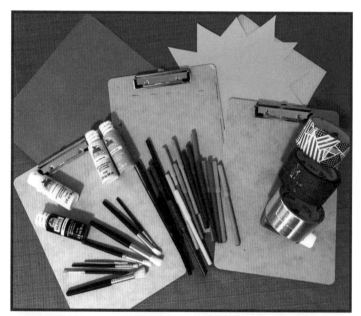

- Plain clipboards
- Covering to decorate the clipboard
  - contact paper
  - duct tape
  - paints and brushes
  - magic markers
- Download and print text, favorite verses, sayings and messages
- Glue stick
- Mod Podge for finishing touches
- Stencils
- Stamping supplies

DIRECTIONS:

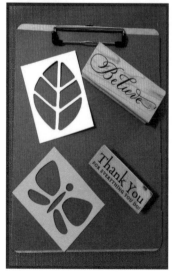
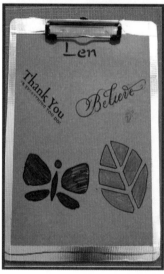

- Decorate your clipboard with the supplies suggested.
- Print the Loved One's name on the board.
- After decorating use Mod Podge to protect your decorations.

NOTE TO CAREGIVER:

- The decorated clipboard can be used to hold coloring projects, family pictures, game sheets or given as presents to friends or grandchildren.

MESSAGE ROCKS

Go on a hunt for flat rocks, clean them, paint them and give them as gifts. What a fun activity to do together with the Loved One.

SAFETY PRECAUTION!

✓ Be aware of the Loved One wandering as you go on your hunt!

SUPPLIES:

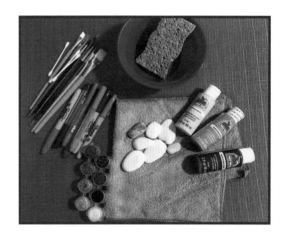

- Flat and smooth rocks
- Water, dish scrubber, towel
- Permanent markers or acrylic paints and brushes
- Mod Podge and brush to seal painting
  (Walmart, Target, Michaels, etc.)

DIRECTIONS:

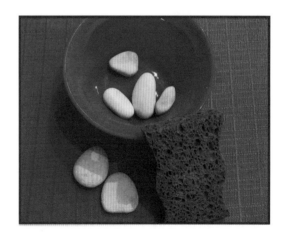

- Wash and dry rocks completely.
- Paint anything on the rocks with markers or acrylic paint.
- Add single words or text with the permanent markers.
- When paint and markers are dry, apply 1-2 coats of Mod Podge to seal your work.

NOTE TO CAREGIVER:

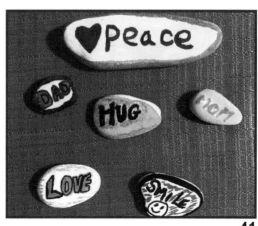

- The rocks can be hidden outside for others to find.
- This is definitely a "feel good" activity. It will bring smiles to anyone who finds the rocks!

FABRIC MARKER ART

Drawing, coloring, stenciling and tracing on fabric can be fun, easy, inexpensive and rewarding.

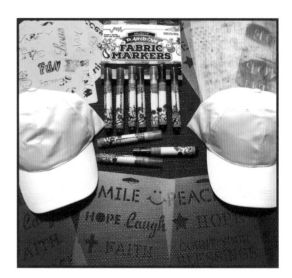

SUPPLIES:

- Various colored fabric markers purchased at a craft store or craft department in a box store such as Walmart
- Fabrics such as:
  - T shirts
  - Hats
  - Sneakers
  - Pieces of fabric (light colored)
- Stencil (s) or item (s) to trace
- Pencil
- Scotch Tape

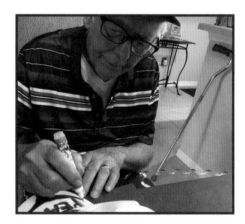

DIRECTIONS:

- Draw designs on a fabric, with the pencil, for the Loved One to color.
- Cut out an item to trace or use a stencil to outline a design on the fabric.
- If helpful consider taping the stencil or cut out on the fabric to hold it in place while sketching the design.
- Have the Loved One apply the color to the fabric.
- After done coloring, wait at least 24 hours, machine wash the fabric on gentle cycle and tumble dry on low.

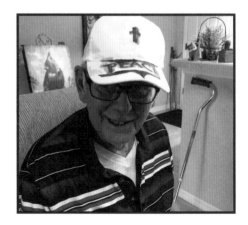

NOTE TO CAREGIVER:

- The Loved One does not have to finish "the coloring" in one sitting. A little at a time works as well.

SAND ART

SAFETY PRECAUTION!

✓ Take care with the use of glass containers, small objects and sand. All are potential hazards to the Loved One.

SUPPLIES:

- Clear plastic or glass bottle or jar with a secure top
- Colored sand
- Paper homemade funnel
- Spoon
- If desired other objects such as stones, shells, etc.
- Tape or glue gun

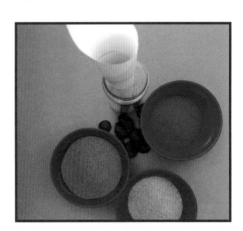

DIRECTIONS:

- Place funnel into the container.
- Spoon in colored sand, one color at a time.
- If desired as you spoon in the sand tilt the container to get a swirl design.
- Change colors and repeat the process until the container is full.
- Seal the top with a cap secured with tape or glue.

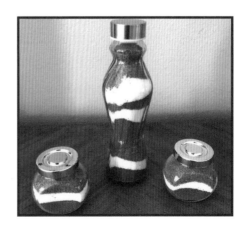

NOTE TO CAREGIVER:

- Colored sand can be purchased inexpensively from a dollar type store.

DECORATING HATS

Just For Fun

There are many ways to do this activity and many reasons to decorate and use a "new" hat: a party for two, a birthday party, anniversary or other celebratory event. Some Loved Ones in their late stage of the illness may not be able to participate in the process of making the hat but thoroughly enjoy the activity and have a lot of fun wearing their hat!

SUPPLIES:

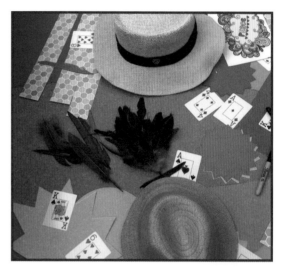

- Low cost hats are easy to find and use for this activity (Dollar Stores, Walmart, etc.)
- Card stock
- Playing cards
- Stickers
- Ribbon
- Magic markers
- Blunt nose scissors
- Scotch tape
- Various colors and designed duct tape
- Stapler
- Feathers

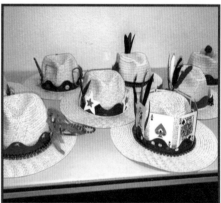

DIRECTIONS:

- Take the card stock and cut it into different sizes and shapes to be attached to the hat later.
- Decorate the card stock with magic markers and stickers.
- In various ways, staple the decorated card stock and playing cards to the hat.
- Consider additionally stapling feathers to the hat.
- Add ribbons and stickers.

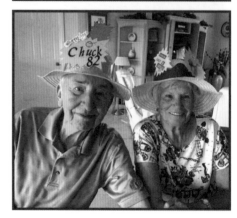

NOTE TO CAREGIVER:

- Your imagination as to various ways of expanding on this activity is limitless.

FOAM STICKERS AND MORE

Make cards, signs, simple posters or decorate with stickers.

SUPPLIES:

• Foam sticker sheets
• Foam (or regular) stickers of all designs and types
• Stickers with numbers and letters
• Foam stickers craft kits
• Greeting cards with blank space inside
  - Birthday
  - Thank you
  - Anniversary
  - Holiday
• Colored card stock
• Plain or colored copy paper

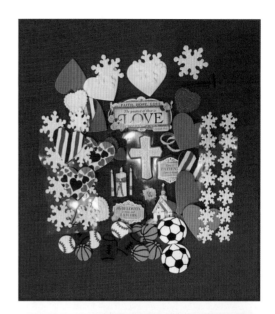

DIRECTIONS:
ACTIVITY NO. 1 GREETING CARDS

• Make a personalized greeting card.

  - Select a card with a lot of blank space for stickers.

  - Talk with the Loved One about whom to give the card and what might be said or shown by the sticker placement.

  - The caregiver can peel off the sticker backing and hand it to the Loved One for placement wherever they want.

  - If the dexterity of the Loved One is not sufficient to handle a sticker, the caregiver can place the sticker and ask The Loved One to tap, tap, tap it into place.

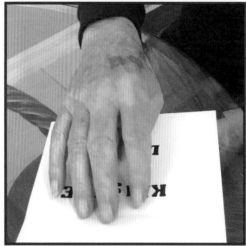

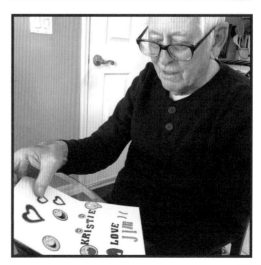

DIRECTIONS:
ACTIVITY NO. 2 DIRECTION SIGNS

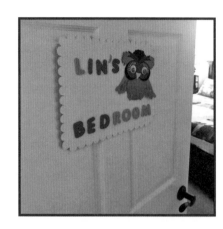

- Make direction signs.

  - (One of the memories that stays a long time with the Loved One may be the ability to read. The Loved One can make direction signs that will assist them in the home. Examples include: Bathroom, Bedroom, Stop Do Not Enter, etc.)

  - As a reference for the Loved One draft out, on a sheet of paper, what the signs will say.

  - Select the largest block letters you can find.

  - Lay out the letters for the Loved One to pick.

  - Peel and have the Loved One place and/or tap in place.

DIRECTIONS:
ACTIVITY NO. 3 DECORATING WITH STICKERS

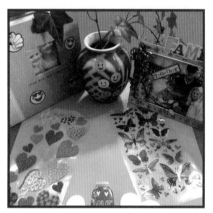

- Just for fun, stick stickers on a piece of paper, family picture frame, photo album, flower pot or other items. You can follow a theme for a holiday, a topic of interest to the Loved One such as sports, birds or flowers, or just to decorate.

  - You also can place stickers on things like glass doors to make them more visible.

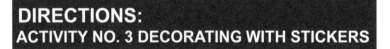

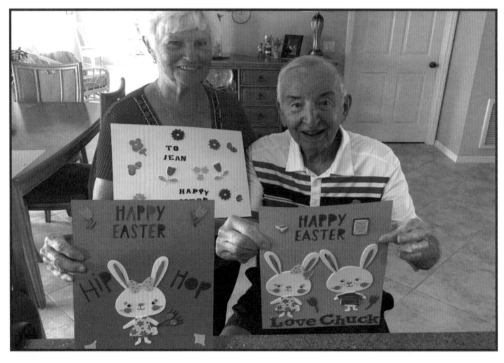

NOTE TO CAREGIVER:

- Even the process of shopping for stickers, on line or in the store is enjoyable for the Loved One.

TABLET ART

This shared activity is not only enjoyable for the Loved One, but the caregiver will also enjoy the process. It is simple, beautiful and enjoyable.

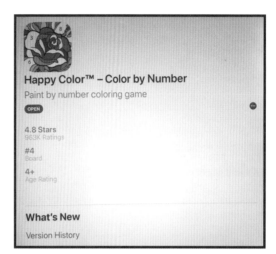

SUPPLIES:

- A tablet (iPad)
- A computer application on art
- Internet service

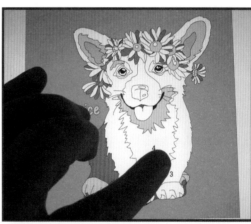

DIRECTIONS:

- Open up your tablet.
- Go to a search engine such a Google.
- Type in free adult computer coloring books.
- Before sharing this activity the caregiver should try out a variety of applications and choose those that are the most workable for the Loved One.
- One feature that all applications possess is the ability to enlarge only a small part of the art piece to easily touch and color.
- Some suggested applications: Paint by Numbers Coloring Book, Bible Coloring & Coloring Games.

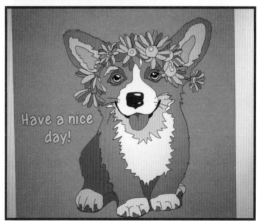

NOTE TO CAREGIVER:

- This activity is worth the effort. If you are not tablet "literate" or have no technical ability get a neighbor or friend to show you how.

*All pictures in this activity are from Happy Color - Color by Number

MAKING A CEREAL BOX NOTEBOOK

In general, this project is for the caregiver to do. The Loved One may really enjoy watching and talking, but their participation may be limited.

SAFETY PRECAUTION!
✓ Keep any sharp objects safely away from the Loved One while doing this project.

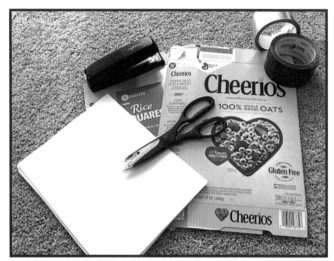

SUPPLIES:

• Scissors
• Stapler
• Cereal box (large)
• Pen
• Duct tape
• Art supplies
• Magic markers
• Paper 8 ½" x 11" (16 to 20 sheets)

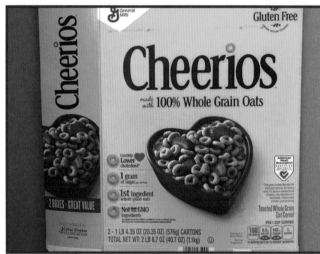

DIRECTIONS:

• Open the top and bottom of the cereal box.

• Cut the box along the middle of the side of the box.

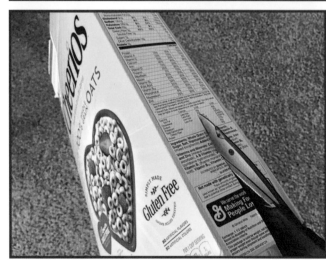

Making a Cereal Box Notebook

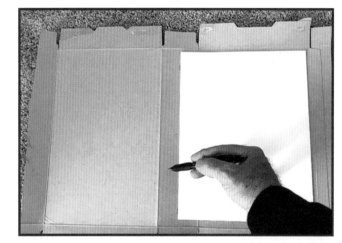

- Open up the box and lay it out, cover side down so the box is flat on a hard surface.
- Layout the paper pages on the right side of the box up to the middle of the other side panel.

- With a pen draw a line along the paper edge up and down the side panel. Remove paper.
- Fold the box along the line you just made.

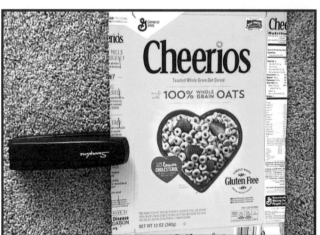

- Open it up and lay out paper just as before.
- While keeping the pages aligned, carefully close the cardboard along your folded line.
- Staple along the fold, evenly spaced from one end to the other making sure the staple goes through the card board and paper.

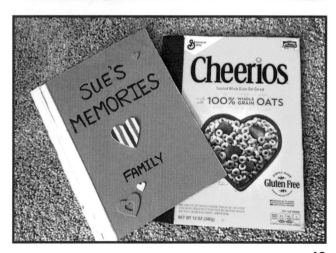

- Apply duct tape along the seam to cover the staples. Decorate as desired.

NOTE TO CAREGIVER:

- Notebooks can be used for pictures the Loved One likes of family, pets, hobbies or sports, or as gifts.

THINGS TO DO WITH...CEREAL BOXES

Don't throw out your cereal boxes until you have tried some of these activities!
They are free, skill building, and fun to make and play!

SAFETY PRECAUTION!

✓ Supervise the Loved One when using blunt scissors.

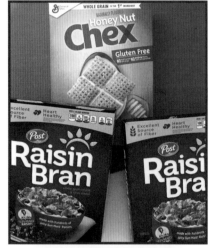

SUPPLIES:

- Cereal Boxes
  - 2 or more of the same cereal box
  - assortment of different cereals
- Children's blunt scissors

DIRECTIONS:
ACTIVITY NO. 1 MATCH GAME

- Play a match game with the fronts of the cereal boxes.

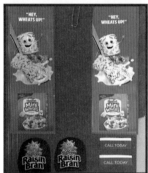

DIRECTIONS:
ACTIVITY NO. 2 I SPY

- Play "I Spy" games for example:
  - find the corn chex, find the corn kernals.

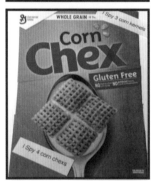

DIRECTIONS:
ACTIVITY NO. 3 PUZZLE

- Make puzzles
- Cut the front of the box into puzzle pieces, the number and size depends on the skill level of the Loved One.

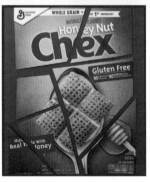

NOTE TO CAREGIVER:

- For more ideas: https://www.pinterest.com/InnerChildFun/made-from-cereal-boxes/

INK BLOT PAINTING!

A Very Easy Version!

This activity can be done with items from your kitchen. It's fun to watch the color spread through the paper towels… looks like magic! Try it and see!

SAFETY PRECAUTION!

✓ Food coloring isn't poisonous, but you don't want the Loved One to drink it. Always be with the Loved One in the kitchen during this activity.

SUPPLIES:

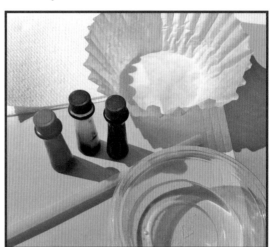

- Plastic protector for work surface
- A straw or eye dropper
- Food coloring or paint (water colors)
- Paper towels or coffee filters
- Water
- Several bowls

DIRECTIONS:

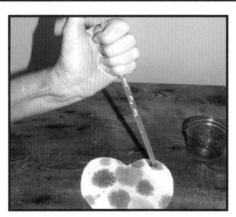

- Put a few drops of food coloring into a bowl with a small amount of water. Use several bowls with different colors.
- Dip the straw into the colored water.
- Hold your finger tight over the top of the straw.
- Keep your finger on the top of the straw, remove the straw from the bowl, and hold the straw over the paper towel or coffee filter.
- Release your finger from the top of the straw and watch the colored water drop onto the paper towel and spread out.
- Do this several times to make a design.

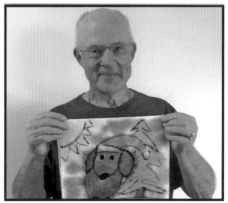

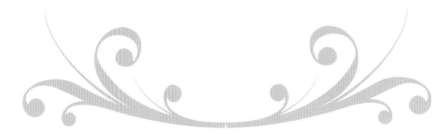

"In life's toughest
moments, our faith will
make all the difference.
God will see us through"

– Allen Hunt
Dreams for your Grandchild

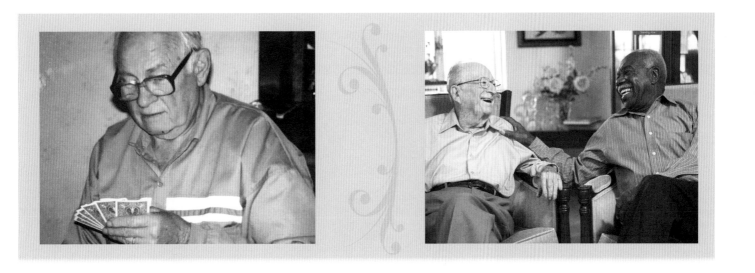

*S*imple
*A*ctivities

LITTLE
OR
NO INSTRUCTION
REQUIRED

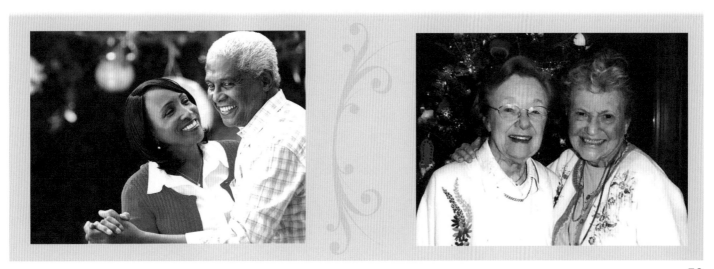

NO INSTRUCTIONS REQUIRED

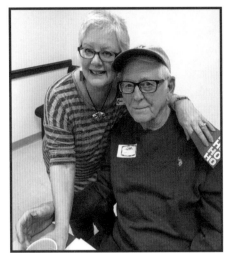
Hugging

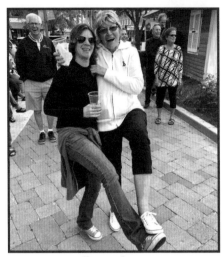
Dancing

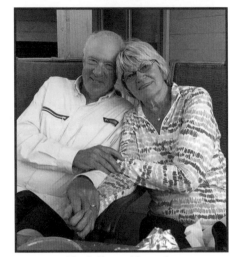
Holding Hands

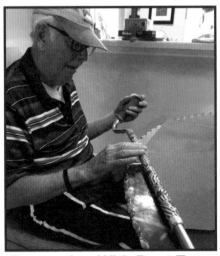
Decorating With Duct Tape

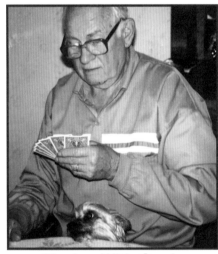
Playing With Cards

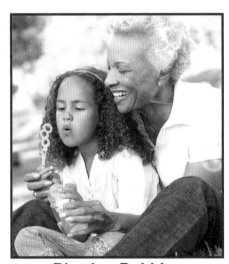
Blowing Bubbles

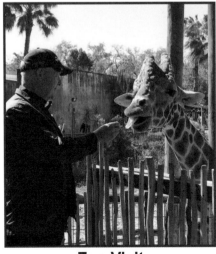
Zoo Visit

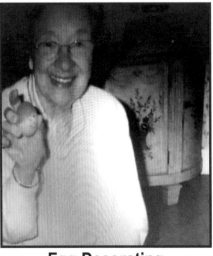
Egg Decorating

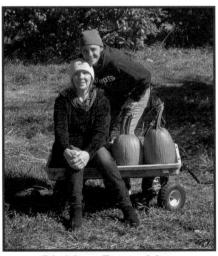
Picking Pumpkins

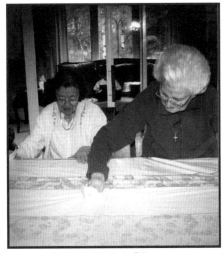

Household Chores

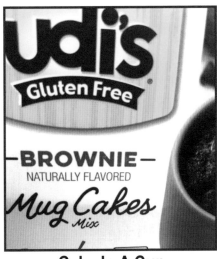

Cake In A Cup

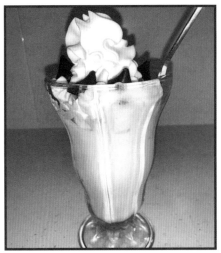

Make A Sundae

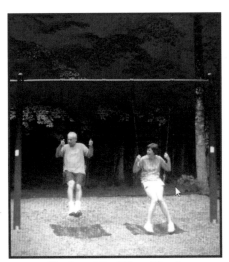

Going To The Park

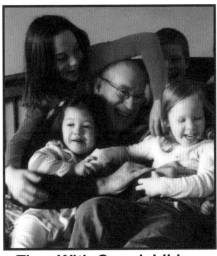

Time With Grandchildren

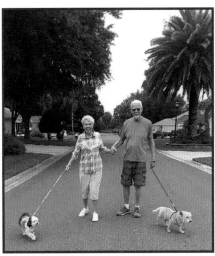

Walk The Dog

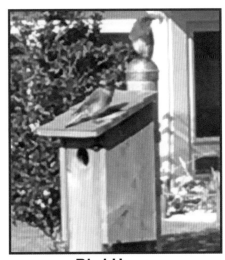

Bird House

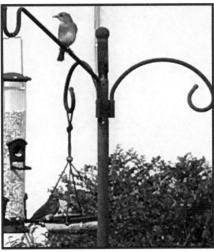

Bird Feeder

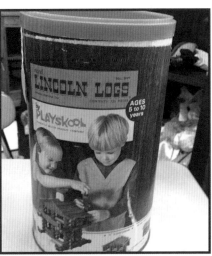

Lincoln Logs

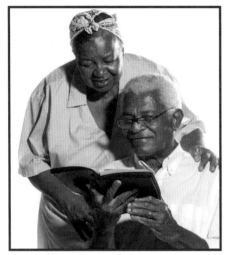

Reading Out Loud

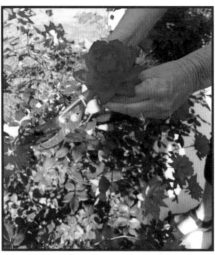

Cutting & Arranging Flowers

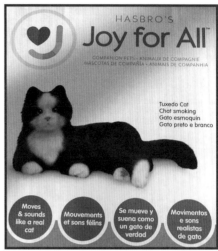

Mechanical Life Like Cat

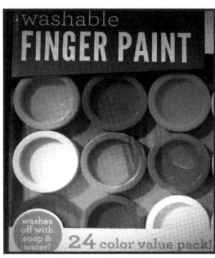

Finger Painting

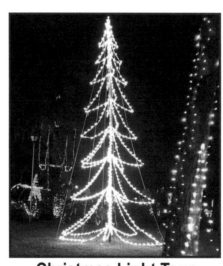

Christmas Light Tour

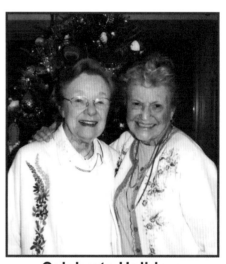

Celebrate Holidays

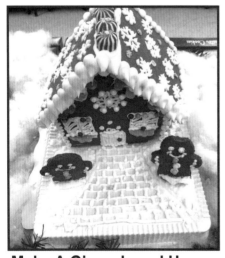

Make A Gingerbread House

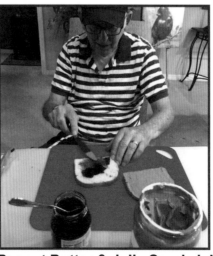

Peanut Butter & Jelly Sandwich

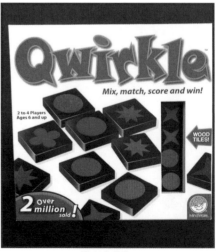

Qwirkle

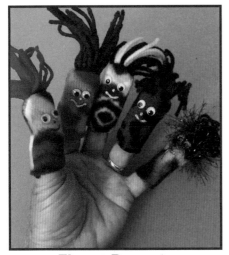

Finger Puppets

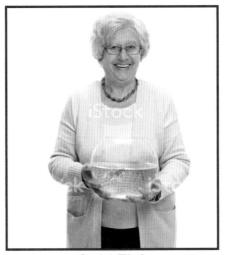

Gold Fish

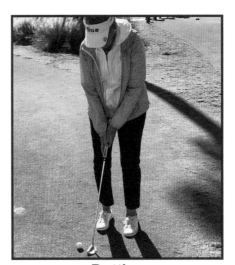

Putting

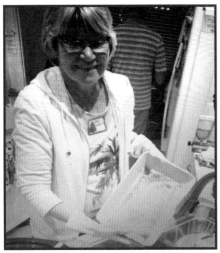

Washing Dishes

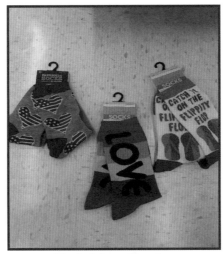

Matching Socks

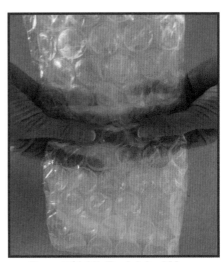

Pop 5/16" Bubble Wrap

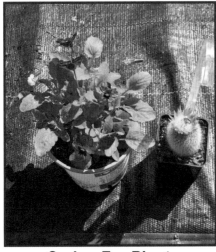

Caring For Plants

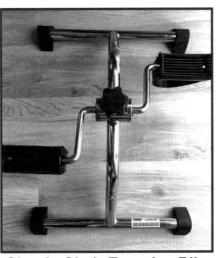

Simple Chair Exercise Bike

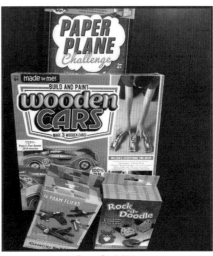

Craft Kits

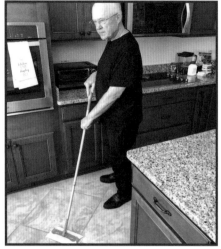

Swiffering

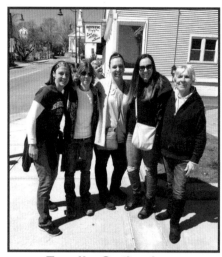

Family Gatherings

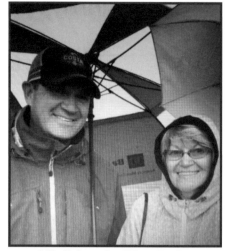

Walking In The Rain

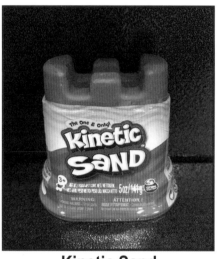

Kinetic Sand

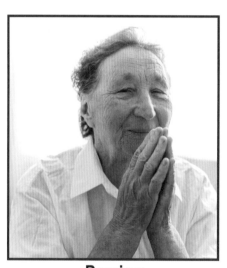

Praying

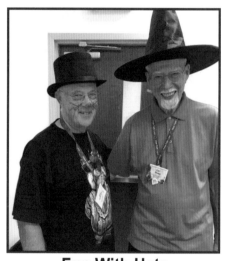

Fun With Hats

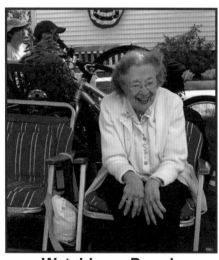

Watching a Parade

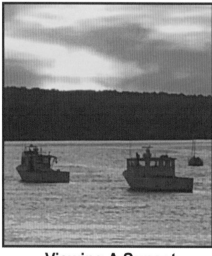

Viewing A Sunset

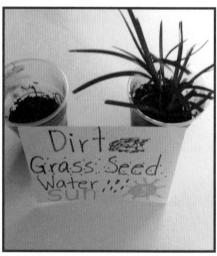

Watching Grass Grow

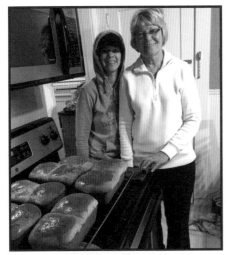
Baking Bread

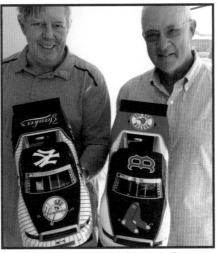
Playing With Model Cars

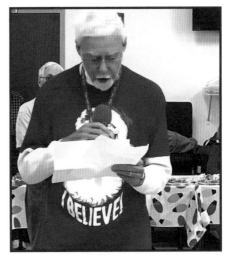
Knock Knock Jokes

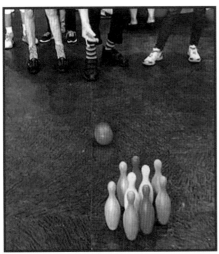
Bowling

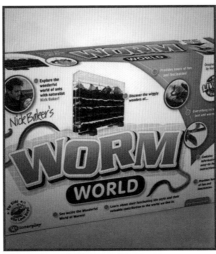
Worm Farm

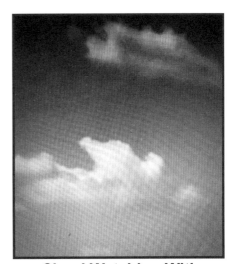
Cloud Watching With Imagination

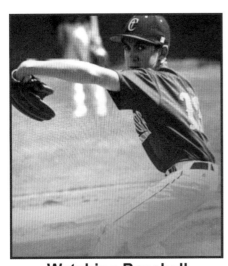
Watching Baseball

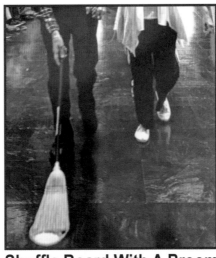
Shuffle Board With A Broom

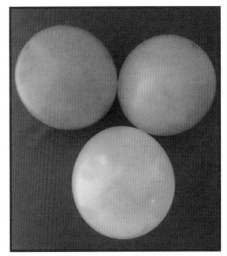
Hitting Balloons

THINGS TO DO WITH PAPER

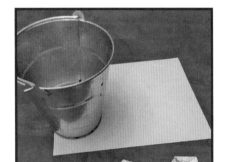

Crumbled Paper in Basket

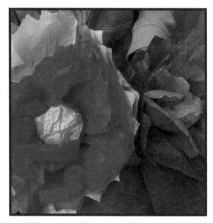

Tissue Paper Flowers

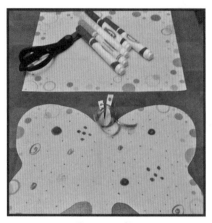

Butterfly

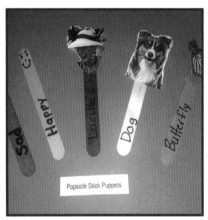

Popsicle Stick Poppers

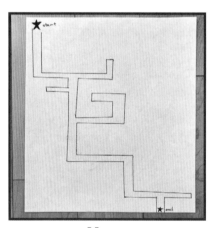

Maze

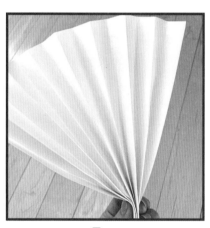

Fan

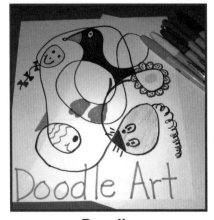

Doodle

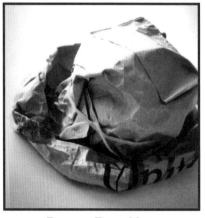

Paper Bag Hat

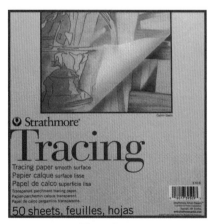

Tracing

Things To Do With Paper 2

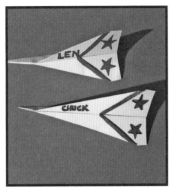
Airplanes

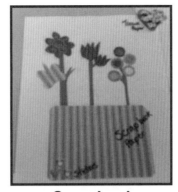
Scrapbook

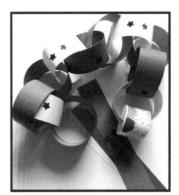
Chains

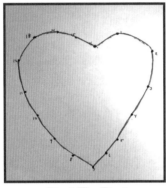
Dot To Dot

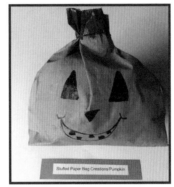
Stuffed Paper Bag

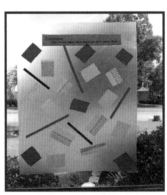
Suncatcher

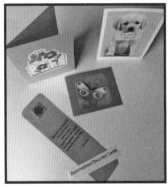
Bookmarks

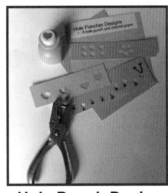
Hole Punch Design

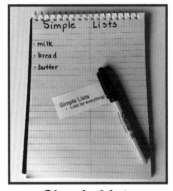
Simple Lists

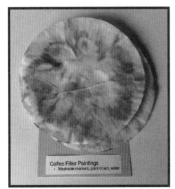
Coffee Filter Painting

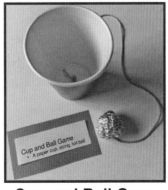
Cup and Ball Game

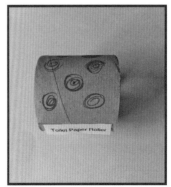
Toilet Paper Roller

ITEMS TO MAKE WITH PAPER PLATES

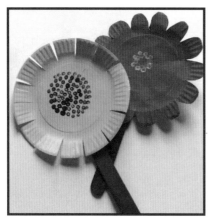
Flower

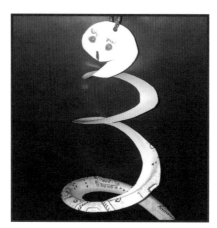
Caterpillar

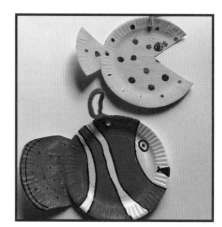
Fish

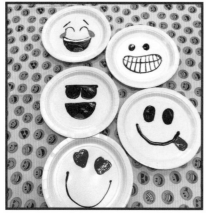
Happy Faces

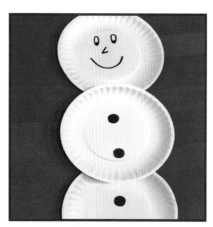
Snowman

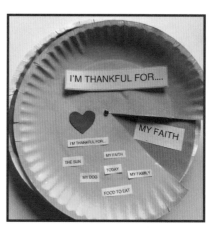
Thankful

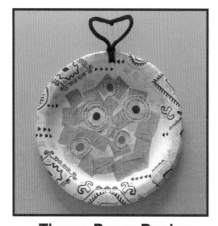
Tissue Paper Design

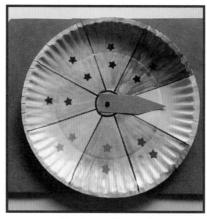
Color Wheel

ENJOYABLE BIRD FEEDERS

There are a few different options when it comes to making bird feeders and a bird bath. If you do not want to make one, then buy one and place it where the Loved One can easily spend hours watching the birds. Just be patient as it may take several days for birds to find the new source of food and water.

SAFETY PRECAUTION!

✓ With some options you may be utilizing implements which pose a danger to the Loved One such as a hot glue gun. Never let the Loved One utilize these implements. Also, bird seed may look good to eat, but it is only for the birds. Supervise well.

ACTIVITY NO. 1
CUP AND SAUCER BIRD FEEDER AND BATH

Do you have old cups and saucers (or plates and small bowls) around the house? The birds will love the baths and feeders you can make from these items.

SUPPLIES:

• Cup, saucer, small bowl or dish from your cabinet or Dollar Tree

• Hot glue gun

• Outdoor table or stand

• Birdseed

• Watercolor

DIRECTIONS:

• Choose a cup, saucer, small bowl or dish.

• Using a hot glue gun attach the cup to the saucer.

• Fill either the cup with bird seed and the saucer with water (or the opposite).

• Place on a table or stand outside so the Loved One can watch the birds "in action".

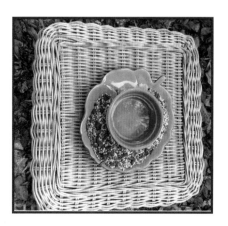

ACTIVITY NO. 2
PINE CONE BIRD FEEDER

Simple and Quick To Make

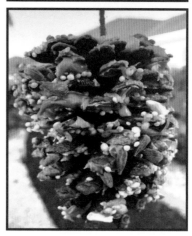

SUPPLIES:

- Pine Cones
- Peanut butter
- Bird seed
- String or ribbon
- Blunt nose scissors
- Plastic spoon and knife
- Plastic table cover

DIRECTIONS:

- Cover the pine cone completely with peanut butter using the plastic knife and spoon.
- Make sure you press the peanut butter firmly into the cracks.
- Spread small piles of bird seed on the plastic table cover.
- Roll the pine cone in the bird seed to cover all around the cone.
- Attach a string and hang on a tree branch in sight of a window in your house.

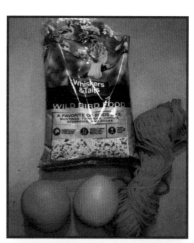

ACTIVITY NO. 3
ORANGE CUP BIRD FEEDER

How simple can you get?

SAFETY PRECAUTION!

✓ The cutting of the orange should only be done by the caregiver.

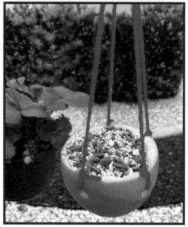

SUPPLIES:

- An orange
- String
- Bird seed
- Plastic knife and spoon

DIRECTIONS:

- With the plastic knife the caregiver should cut the orange in half.
- Scoop the fruit out of the orange with the plastic knife and spoon.
- Attach string to the orange.
- Add bird seed.
- Hang the bird feeder outside.

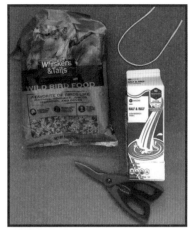

ACTIVITY NO. 4
MILK CARTON BIRD FEEDER

SAFETY PRECAUTION!
✓ The cutting of the feeder openings should only be done by the caregiver.

SUPPLIES:

- Empty milk carton
- String
- Scissors
- Glass safe suction cup hook (option)

DIRECTIONS:

- The caregiver should cut out opening as shown.
- Attach string.
- Fill with seed and hang.

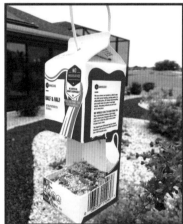

NOTE TO CAREGIVER:

- As an option you can place a glass safe suction hook on the outside of a window and hang the milk carton feeder from it thereby permitting the Loved One to see feeding birds up close.

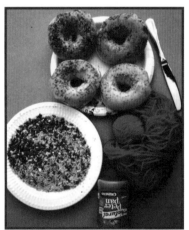

ACTIVITY NO. 5
BAGEL BIRD FEEDERS

SUPPLIES:

- Bagels
- Peanut butter
- Bird seed
- Plastic knife and spoon
- String

DIRECTIONS:

- Cut the bagels in half. This process is to be done only by the caregiver.
- Completely cover the flat side of the bagel with peanut butter.
- Dip or press the peanut butter side of the bagel on to a plate of bird seed.
- Tie the string through the hole in the bagel. Hang outside.

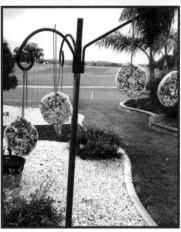

ACTIVITY NO. 6
CHEERIO BIRD FEEDER

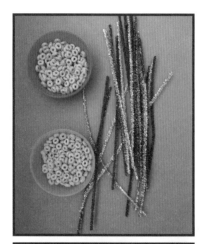

SUPPLIES:

• Pipe cleaners
• Cheerios

DIRECTIONS:

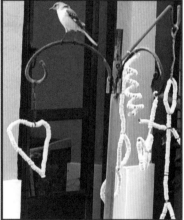

• At one end of a pipe cleaner twist it into a loop so the Cheerios will not pass.

• Thread Cheerios onto the remainder of the pipe cleaner.

• Leave some of the pipe cleaner at the end.

• Attach it to the other end of the cleaner, another cleaner or just twist the top and make it in to a hanger.

• Shape or twist as desired.

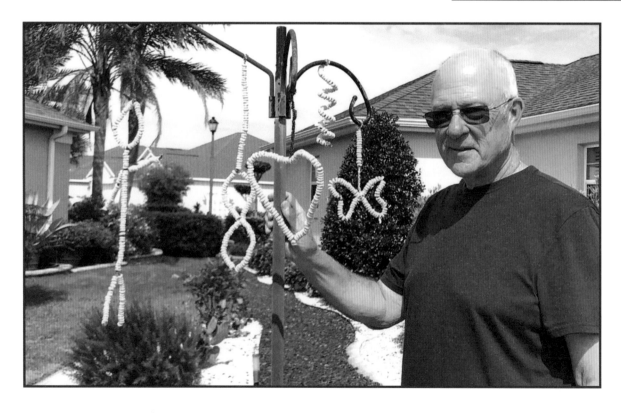

NOTE TO CAREGIVER:

• This is the simplest of all the feeders and no matter how they are made they all look like works of art.

PIPE FITTING

SAFETY PRECAUTION!

✓ Simply fit pieces of pipe together and take them apart..

SUPPLIES:

- 4 or more 6' sections of PVC pipe
- 10 or more PVC couplings
- 10 or more PVC elbows
- Pipe cutter
- Storage container

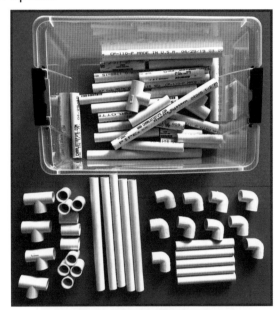

DIRECTIONS:

- Before working with the Loved One cut the 6' sections of PVC pipe into numerous smaller pieces.

- Place them into the storage container for easy access by the Loved One.

- The caregiver can start by connecting 2 pipe sections with a coupling

- The Loved One can continue with or without assistance to assemble all or many of the pipe sections.

- The caregiver can take cell phone pictures of the assembled sections.

- When the Loved One is no longer interested in assembling sections, it's time to have fun taking it all apart and putting the pieces back into the storage container.

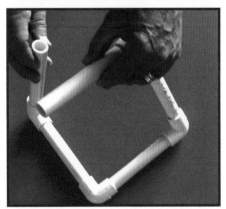

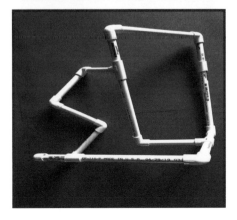

NOTE TO CAREGIVER:

- Your imagination to ways to expand the activity is limitless. One idea is to make and hang signs from the assembled pipes.

PRAYER BOX

Fun to make and a comfort to have

SUPPLIES:

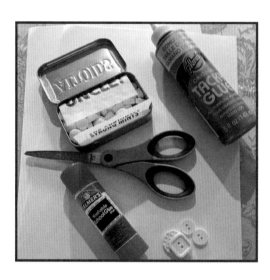

- Altoids box
- White computer paper
- Glue stick
- Tacky glue
- Computer & printer
- Decorative buttons

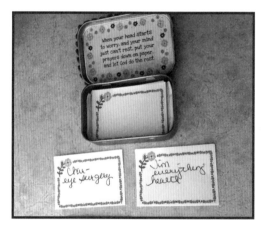

DIRECTIONS:

- Empty the Altoids box.
- On the computer, type words in text boxes, for example:
  - Pray More Worry Less
  - When your head starts to worry and your mind can't rest, put your prayers down and let God do the rest.
- Print out words and cut out.
- Glue words on top of lid and underside of lid.
- Decorate with buttons, etc. as you like.
- Write prayers on small rectangles of paper that fit in the box.

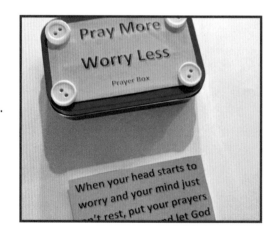

NOTE TO CAREGIVER:

- The prayer box is easy to carry with you wherever you go. Let the Loved One pick out a prayer and read it together.

SOCK WARMERS

Cold hands, frozen toes, a tummy ache, a warm snuggler … sock warmers are just for you and the Loved One to make and use! This is an easy gift idea as well!

SAFETY PRECAUTION!

✓ Be sure and stay with the Loved One while doing this activity. The rice is edible but raw rice may cause stomach aches if a quantity of rice is ingested. After making the sock warmer, test the time in the microwave so your sock isn't too hot to touch.

SUPPLIES:

- Socks – colorful tube or knee socks
  - Dollar Tree, Walmart or ones you already have
- Uncooked rice
- Funnel
  - Dollar Tree or homemade with card stock

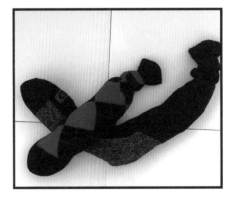

DIRECTIONS:

- Using a funnel, fill a tube sock or knee sock with rice.
- Fill 2/3 full, leaving room to tie a tight knot at the opening of the sock.
- When ready to use, put in the microwave for 30 plus seconds to warm it up.
- Because of its long shape, it's perfect for laying across stomachs, on limbs and across the back of your neck.

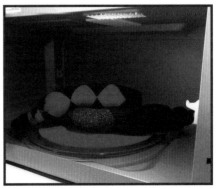

NOTE TO CAREGIVER:

- You can also use smaller socks, fill with rice, and use as bean bags, tossing them back and forth to each other.

STAMPING WITH PENCIL ERASERS

Make your own stamp pads using pencil erasers and create beautiful pictures together with the Loved One.

SAFETY PRECAUTION!

✓ Watch for paint and pencils going into mouths! Supervise! Use washable paint in case it gets on other items.

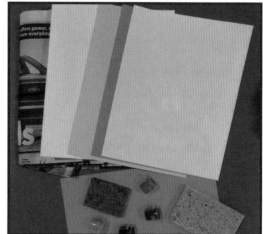

SUPPLIES:

- Inexpensive sponges
- Small plastic containers for each sponge
- Poster paint
- Cardstock or canvas board
- Optional: plain gift boxes, white wrapping paper
- Pencils with erasers on end
- Water and paper towels for cleanup
- Old newspapers for table protection

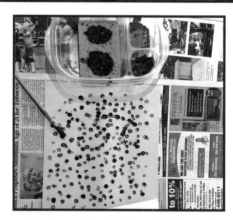

DIRECTIONS:

- Prepare your work space with newspapers.
- Lay out paper/item you will paint.
- Cut sponges to fit plastic containers.
  - One sponge per container.
- Dampen sponges with a little water.
- Dab paint onto sponge.
  - Use a different paint per sponge.
- Work paint into sponge.
- Using the eraser on the end of a pencil, dab the painted sponge and then dab the paper.
  - Use a different pencil for each color or wipe eraser clean after each paint.
- Make a design of choice.

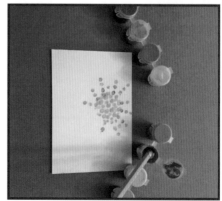

NOTE TO CAREGIVER:

- Depending on the skills of the Loved One, you can draw a simple picture, or print one from the internet, and let the Loved One dab the painted eraser onto a picture rather than make a design.

JEANNE'S BUTTON ACTIVITY

Jeanne created this activity for her Loved One, Chuck, and it became one of his favorites.

SAFETY PRECAUTION!

✓ As most buttons are small this is a 1 to 1 person activity which requires the caregiver's participation and supervision.

SUPPLIES:

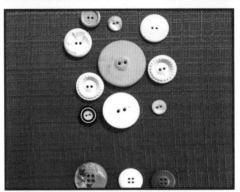

- Plenty of old buttons
- Container to store the buttons
- 6 small plastic bowls
  (all different colors if possible)
- Notecards or Post-it Notes to label the bowls accordingly.

DIRECTIONS:

- Jeanne often sorted the buttons with Chuck, in some of the following ways:
  - Dark colors
  - Light colors
  - Flat buttons
  - Raised buttons
  - 4 Hole buttons
  - 2 Hole buttons
- Label the bowls appropriately.
- Depending on the Loved One's skill level:
  - The caregiver can select a button and ask the Loved One in which bowl the button should be placed.
  - The Loved One can also select a button and make the decision on their own where the button belongs.

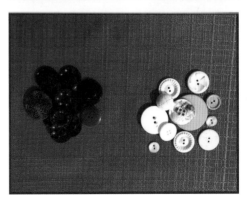

NOTE TO CAREGIVER:

- Antique centers and friends are a great source to acquire a variety of buttons.

SHAVING CREAM ART

Easy to do, fun activity with little preparation time.

SAFETY PRECAUTION!

✓ This activity should be done in the kitchen area and near the sink. Make sure you have all your supplies at the table before you start. The caregiver will not want to leave the table before the complletition of the activity.

SUPPLIES:

• Glass top table

• Plenty of terry cloth towels

• Some paper towels

• Men's shaving cream
  (Not menthol shaving cream)

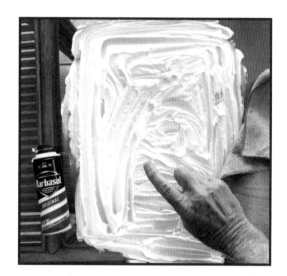

DIRECTIONS:

• This activity should be done with the Loved One seated at the table.

• Take the shaving cream and spread it out on the glass top table to any size or shape you desire. The Loved One will enjoy this!

• Wipe off your hands with the towel as often as needed.

• With your fingers, draw, doodle, or scribble on the shaving cream "till your heart's content!"

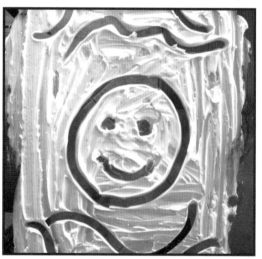

NOTE TO CAREGIVER:

• Cleaning up is easy. You will need more terry cloth towels than you think.

FAMILY DRY ERASE MESSAGE BOARD

Stage Appropriate:
Early & Middle

Number of Participants:
1 to 1

A Family Message Board is a great visual reminder of important things about each day! You and the Loved One can work on it together, talk about important days, family photos and personalize it as much as you want.

SAFETY PRECAUTION!

✓ Be sure to supervise the Loved One with the dry erase markers and the glue stick.

SUPPLIES:

- Large picture frame, preferably with Plexiglass (Dollar Tree)
- Dry erase markers
- Colored paper
- Calendar
- Stickers
- Glue stick
- Blunt nose scissors
- Magazines
- Photos

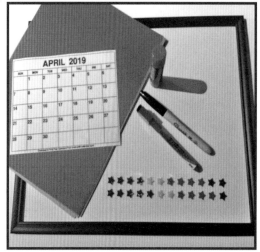

DIRECTIONS:

- Type or write the headings on the colored paper and decorate, or use letters cut out from a magazine.
- Glue headings on the back of the glass.
- Put frame back together.
- Using a dry erase marker, write on top of frame's glass each day.
- Heading suggestions:
  - Our Calendar
  - Our Plans for Today
  - Grocery List
  - Star of the Day (use a picture of a relative or friend)
  - Message of the day

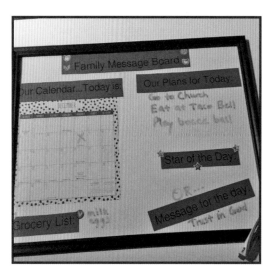

NOTE TO CAREGIVER:

- You can also use this family dry erase message board for many things: to draw and guess pictures and words, to make mazes and to scribble pictures.

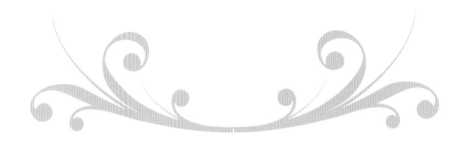

I can do everything through Christ who gives me strength

Phil. 4:13

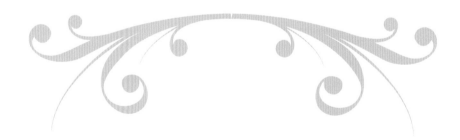

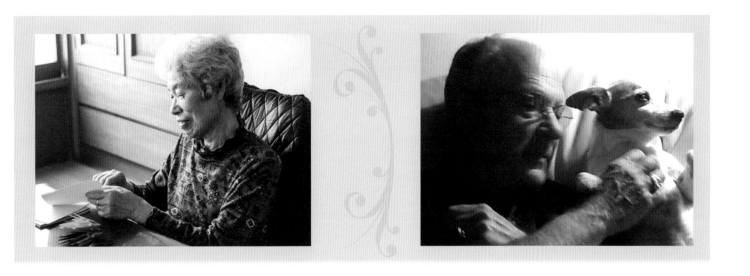

*A*round *T*he *H*ouse

MANY ACTIVITIES CAN BE STRUCTURED WITHIN THE HOUSE
AND WITH ITEMS FOUND AROUND THE HOUSE.

SOME ACTIVITIES ARE JUST FOR ENJOYMENT WHILE
OTHERS ARE ORIENTED TO PROVIDE LOVED ONES
A SENSE OF ACCOMPLISHMENT.

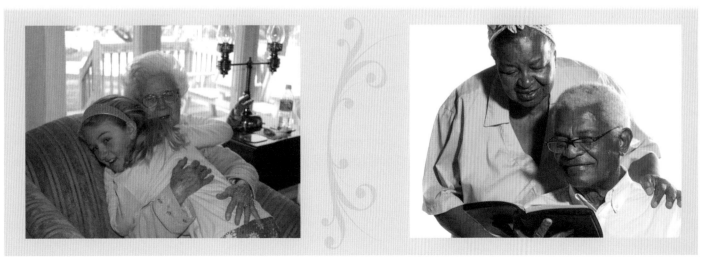

PETS

Any living animal as well as inanimate animals, such as stuffed or mechanical animals, can be a cherished pet and provide hours of enjoyment for the Loved One and caregiver. (Consideration should be given to the additional time and resources care of a pet may have on the already heavy demands of the caregiver.)

SAFETY PRECAUTION!

✓ Care must be taken – pets can be a tripping hazard or may frighten the Loved One.

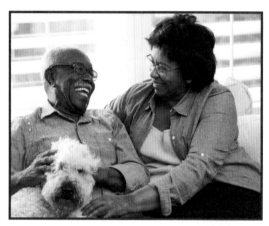

SUPPLIES:

• Pets may include: dogs, cats, tropical fish, birds, rabbits, hamsters and more.

• Accessories to care for pets. Some pet accessories may be costly depending on the type of pet selected.

DIRECTIONS:

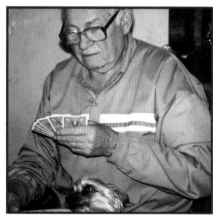

• Consideration should be given to the Loved One's ability to participate in the care and enjoyment of the pet.

• Alternatives to owning a pet should be considered. Alternative considerations include:

 - Taking trips to an animal shelter. Talk with them about what you are doing and ask if there is any volunteer work the Loved One can do. Shelters often care for many kinds of animals other than dogs and cats, that are small, docile and in need of attention.

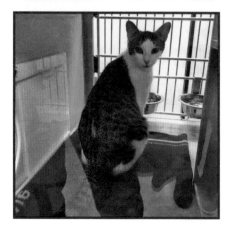

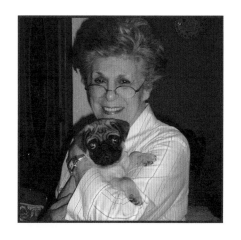

- A neighbor might have a pet that is suitable and has the temperament that will bring joy to the Loved One for short periods of time. They may visit your home or you may visit theirs. Take care to ensure that the pet's behavior and characteristics will not scare or harm the Loved One.

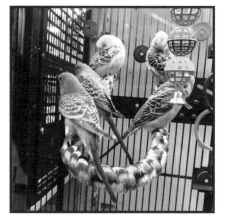

- Take trips to pet stores or zoos. While there, talk about the animals with the Loved One, and take pictures with your phone. Show and talk about the pictures later. You can also make a memory book of your trip with printed photos.

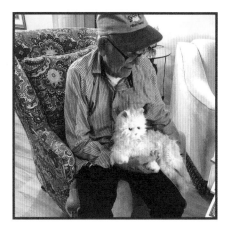

- Many Loved Ones enjoy stuffed, life-like or mechanical animals. There are a number of them on the market developed for individuals with Alzheimer's. Many Loved Ones will treat the model animal as a live pet, caregivers often follow this behavior. It is ok. Enjoy the moment.

NOTE TO CAREGIVER:

• There are wonderful YouTube or Google animal clips you can watch. Just type in the kind of animal you or the Loved One enjoys.

YouTube suggestions include:
- "Kids and dogs bath time."
- "Sweet mama dog interacting with child."
- "Unbelievable unlikely animal friendships."
- "Funny guilty dog compilations."
- "Funny cat compilation."

SURPRISE GIFTS

Fun for Everyone

Stage Appropriate:
Early, Middle & Some Late

Number of Participants:
1 to 3 or more

Most of us enjoy gifts, and surprise gifts are often the best! Loved Ones often enjoy surprise gifts more than most. This activity is one that the caregiver does for the Loved One and not with the Loved One.

SAFETY PRECAUTION!

✓ Many gifts work well as long as they are safe for the Loved One.

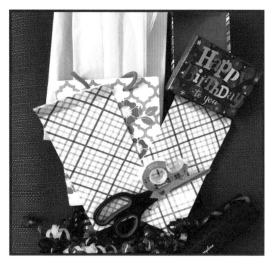

SUPPLIES:

- Gift bags
- Wrapping paper
- Bows
- Scotch tape
- Scissors
- Small gifts, such as crayons, photos, candy, cookies and holiday related items

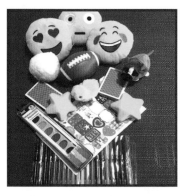

DIRECTIONS:

- Select a gift.
- Wrap the gift simply or as ornately as you wish.
- Share the joy the Loved One gets as they open their gift.

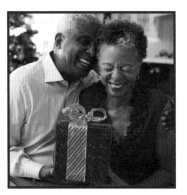
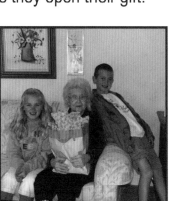
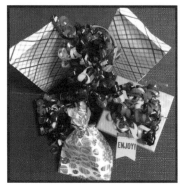

NOTE TO CAREGIVER:

- You can give surprise gifts often. It can be as simple as a cookie. The Loved One may find more joy from the act of receiving the gift than the gift itself.

DVDS

Easy to use and helpful

A great alternative to TV. When the caregiver utilizes DVDs they control what is being watched. The Loved Ones enjoy DVDs because they are not interrupted by commercials.

SAFETY PRECAUTION!

✓ Please avoid DVD topics that contain violence of any type.

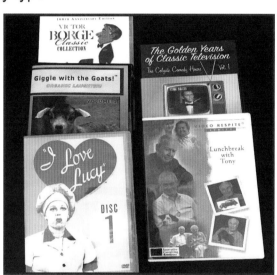

SUPPLIES:

• Computer or DVD player

• DVDs purchased in a store or online. Also check if your local library has a DVD loaner program.

• Some DVD recommended topics include:
  - Victor Borge
  - I Love Lucy
  - Gigglewiththegoats.com
  - Sports
  - Animals
  - Lunch Break with Tony (videorespite.com)

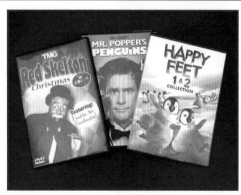

DIRECTIONS:

• Select a DVD and play

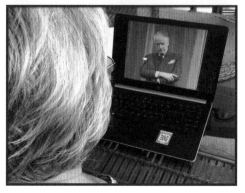

NOTE TO CAREGIVER:

• Avoid children's DVDs. Preview all DVDs prior to playing for the Loved One. You can play the same DVD many times over if it is the Loved One's favorite.

SENSORY PERCEPTION BAG

A sensory activity to do using things from around your house

There are many items around the house that you can put into a decorative bag that the Loved One will enjoy holding one item at a time. Squeezing, stroking and manipulating are activities that could bring the Loved One moments of peace and calm.

SAFETY PRECAUTION!

✓ Be sure to supervise the Loved One when using small items.

SUPPLIES:

• Large gift bag
• Assortment of items from around your house
• Some suggested items:
  - Scarf, silk-like
  - Tie
  - Cotton balls in a Ziploc bag
  - Soft dog toy
  - Scrub sponge
  - Balled up tissue paper
  - Ribbon
  - Soft toys
  - Small plastic container and lid containing smaller objects like a: smooth stone, palm cross, and a large button

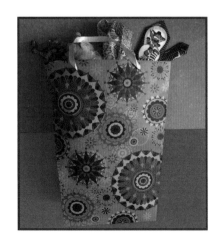

DIRECTIONS:

• Place all the items in the large decorative gift bag.

Sensory Perception Bag 2

- Have the Loved One select one item from the bag.

- Encourage the Loved One to feel, manipulate, rub and move the item through their fingers.

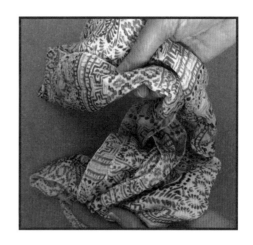

- You may want to show or assist the Loved One in ways to perceive the feeling of the item.

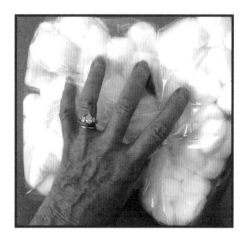

- If the Loved One is disinterested in the item have him/her set it aside and select another item.

- Take your time. As long as the Loved One is interested in holding the item wait before selecting another item.

- Select another item.

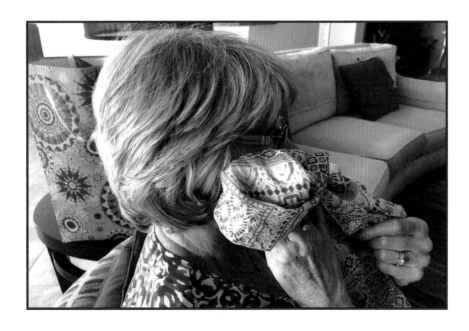

NOTE TO CAREGIVER:

- This is purely a sensory activity for the Loved One to enjoy. It is not unusual for the Loved One to just hold an item for a long time.

YOUTUBE IS YOUR FRIEND

… and similar technology

When utilizing technologies like YouTube the caregiver is controlling the material to be reviewed by the Loved One.

SAFETY PRECAUTION!

✓ Preview all material to insure it is not frightening or contains violence.

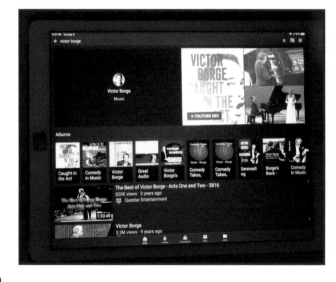

SUPPLIES:

• Computer or Tablet device
• Wi Fi

DIRECTIONS:

• Turn on the device.
• Click on YouTube icon or use a Google type search and type in YouTube.
• When YouTube site comes up click on the magnifying glass at the top right hand corner of the screen.
• Type in the item or topic of interest to be viewed.
• Some suggested topics include:
  - Music comedy
  - Marx Brothers
  - Victor Borge
  - Classical music in the key of comedy
  - Unusual Music
  - Water glasses secret performer
  - Street perform Wintergatan – Marble Machine
  - Piano street performers

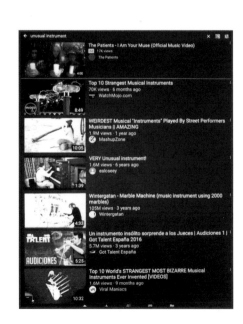

YouTube Is Your Friend 2

- Pets
- Pet animals getting a bath.
- Fun dog tricks with Roque & Ruger

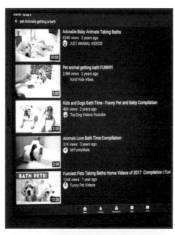

- Grandparents / Kids
- Brian Kinder, Grandma, Grandpa song
- Grandparents day song
- Little big shots by Steve Harvey

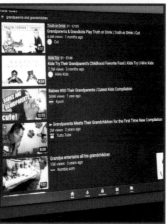

- Sports
- Golf top 10
- Bowling top 10
- Football top 10

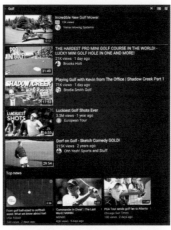

Other ideas to explore:
- Christmas
- Cars
- Dancing/songs
- Old tv comedies, shows, commercials

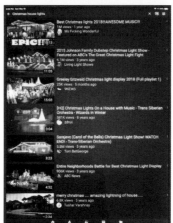

NOTE TO CAREGIVER:
• Enjoy!

SORTING LAUNDRY

Encourages Loved One To Be Helpful

Stage Appropriate:
Early & Middle

Number of Participants:
1 to 1

These are just a few ideas to get you started on a sorting activity. You can modify the activity to match the abilities and interest of the Loved One. You can also create other sorting activities such as flatware, napkins, plastic dishes, cards by color or numbers, etc. Also see activity titled Sorting Coins.

SAFETY PRECAUTION!

✓ If necessary to avoid any tripping or falling hazards, remove large bulky items from the laundry such as, sheets or bathrobes. Preferably have the Loved One sit while sorting.

SUPPLIES:

• Laundry

• Laundry basket

• Safe place for the Loved One to sort (Kitchen table, couch, etc.)

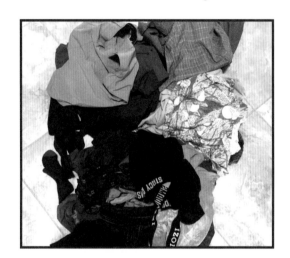

DIRECTIONS:
ACTIVITY NO. 1 SORTING DIRTY CLOTHES

• Have the Loved One look at each piece of clothing and tell or show which pile is dark or light laundry.

• If possible have the Loved One put sorted colors into the washer.

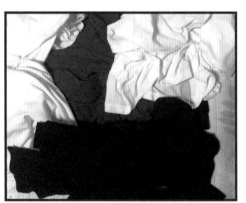

DIRECTIONS:
ACTIVITY NO. 2 SORTING HIS AND HERS

• The clean and dry laundry now can be sorted into "his & hers" piles.

• Hold up a piece of laundry and ask the Loved One if it should be in his or her pile.

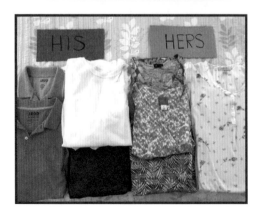

DIRECTIONS:
ACTIVITY NO. 3 MORE SORTING

• Go to the pile of the Loved One.

• Holding up one item of laundry at a time sort like items into like piles. Example – tee shirts into one pile, socks into another.

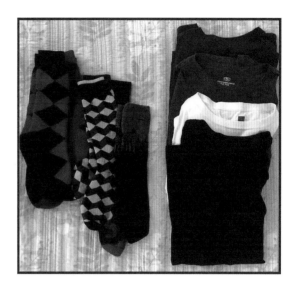

• The Loved One simply tells you by word or gesture which pile to place like items.

• If possible and safe the Loved One can assist the caregiver put their sorted, clean laundry "away".

• At the conclusion of the activity thank the Loved One for her/ his help. This gesture will help validate how important their assistance is to you and show appreciation for their help.

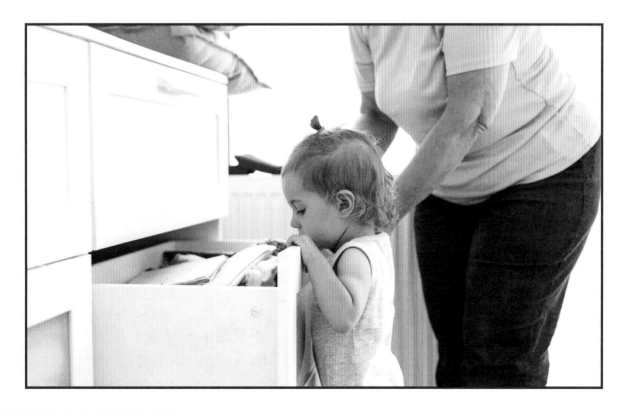

NOTE TO CAREGIVER:

• There is no such thing as a "wrong pile", anything goes. You can always make adjustments later. This could bring all an occasional smile.

PIPE CLEANERS!

Stage Appropriate:
Early to Middle

Number of Participants:
1 to 3

Have you ever thought of fun things to do with pipe cleaners? They are great for fine motor skills, feeling silly, and cheap to buy! Here are a few ideas for this together activity.
https://www.pinterest.com/explore/pipe/cleaners/

SAFETY PRECAUTION!

✓ Watch out for the pipe cleaners going into mouths. The ends have a sharp wire but it can be bent a little or taped to eliminate the sharpness. With supervision, these are fun and easy activities for you and the Loved One.

SUPPLIES:

- Assortment of pipe cleaners
- Old spice jar or Pringles type can
- Colander
- Strong magnet (wand if possible)
- Clear plastic water or soda bottle
- Children's blunt scissors

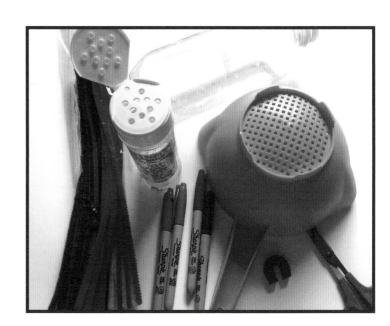

DIRECTIONS: ACTIVITY 1
PIPE CLEANER SORT

- Cut the pipe cleaners in half.
- Use an old spice jar, or Pringles type can.
- With permanent markers, color the holes to match the pipe cleaners.
- Stick the pipe cleaners in the holes.

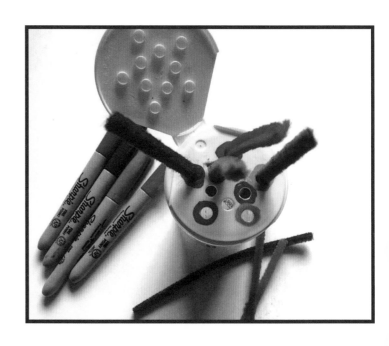

DIRECTIONS: ACTIVITY 2
PIPE CLEANER STICK-UM

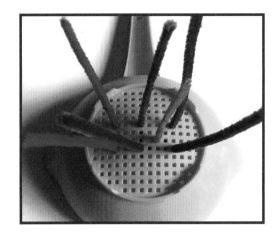

• Use a kitchen colander and stick the pipe cleaners into holes.

• Create a design or just stick into holes.
• It's a win-win activity and great skill building.

DIRECTIONS: ACTIVITY 3
PIPE CLEANER STICK PEOPLE/ANIMALS

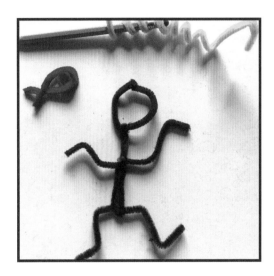

• Bend and twist pipe cleaners to make people/animals/ a design.

• To create wiggle worms, wrap pipe cleaners around a pencil.

• Talk about your silly creation.

DIRECTIONS: ACTIVITY 4
MAGNETIC PIPE CLEANER FUN

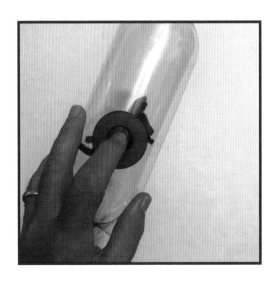

• Cut pipe cleaners into different lengths, 1-2" long and put into an empty water or soda bottle. Secure the lid.

• Place a strong magnet or magnetic wand on the outside of the bottle and move it around to move the pipe cleaners.

• Choose a color to try to move each time.

• It's magic… have fun!

NOTE TO CAREGIVER:

• Playing with pipe cleaners can be very therapeutic… keeping hands busy but constructive. You will no doubt think of other activities to do with pipe cleaners.

SEEK AND FIND

This activity is simple and rewarding for most Loved Ones. It does not require much preparation and can be done at a moment's notice. There are a variety of different ways to carry out this activity depending on the Loved One's interest and abilities.

SAFETY PRECAUTION!

✓ Be aware and take preventive care to insure that the activity does not result in the Loved One tripping or falling. Take precautions as necessary.

SUPPLIES:

• Cellphone or tablet with a camera

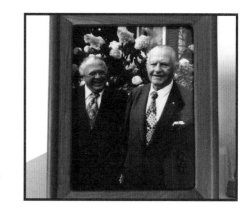

DIRECTIONS:

• Walk around the room with the Loved One. Sitting in a favorite room is also ok.

• Look around the room, point out a single item at a time and talk about it. Items such as a family photo, picture, plant or lamp.

• With your cellphone or tablet camera take a picture of the individual item. Clearly frame the item so the item is all that is in the picture.

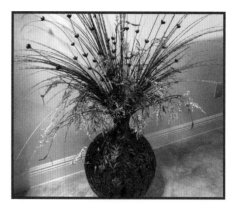

• Once you have completed your photo tour, look at a single photo show it to the Loved One and talk about it.

• Ask the Loved One to look around the room and find the item in the room that matches the photo.

• If the Loved One has difficulty finding the items give hints.

• In some situations it may be necessary to bring the Loved One to the item, place the photo near it and ask: Is this a match- do they look alike?

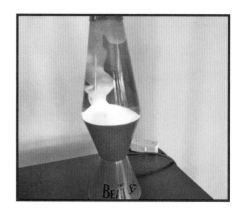

• Whatever the Loved One answers can always be responded to in a positive manner by simply saying " I can see how you answered that way".

NOTE TO CAREGIVER:

• This same activity can be done outside in the yard or driveway while sitting comfortably in a chair.

CUP DECORATING

And Stacking

This activity is easy to do, inexpensive, very popular and enjoyable. Many of us over a long time have enjoyed games where we see how high we can stack something and there has always been someone around that cannot wait to knock the stack down.

SAFETY PRECAUTION!

✓ Only do this activity while the Loved One is sitting down.

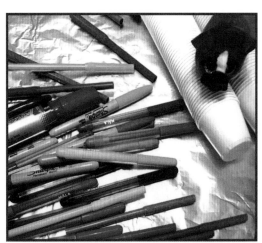

SUPPLIES:

• Any size paper or plastic cup that you can color on with a sharpie, 3 oz. bathroom cups are popular. They can be stacked high and wide in a small space.

• Sharpie or permanent marker

• A flat surface to work on

• Possibly a small very soft toy that if thrown will not hurt anyone or anything.

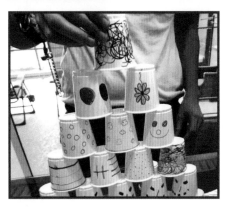

DIRECTIONS:

• Separate the cups and draw a decoration on each cup with a colored permanent marker. Do not be overly concerned with how the Loved One decorates them.

• Decorate as many as you want, 30 cups per person will not be too many.

• Line up 6-8 cups in front of the Loved One on a stable flat surface.

• Let the Loved One start stacking upon the base of 6-8 cups. You may have to start the stacking so the Loved One will see how to stack the cups.

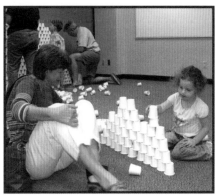

NOTE TO CAREGIVER:

• Once stacked, the Loved One may want to reverse the process and one by one unstack them. This is also enjoyable.

SIFTING THROUGH COINS

SAFETY PRECAUTION!

✓ Coins and small items are choking hazards and may carry harmful germs. Clean coins thoroughly, always supervise the Loved One and put away coins and small objects after the activity for safe keeping. Never use a glass or breakable bowl. Do not heat water on stove – use warm water from the faucet.

SUPPLIES:

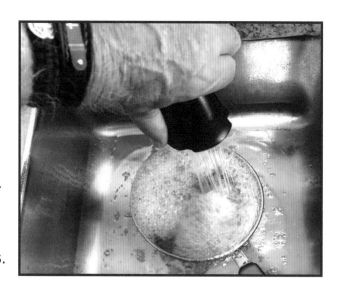

- Coins, religious or novelty coins
- Plastic bowl. Even a clean dog dish is good. Never utilize a glass or breakable bowl.
- Disinfectant such as Lysol
- Rubber gloves
- Paper or cloth towel
- A pot or pan with handle
- Hand sanitizer

DIRECTIONS:

- Using rubber gloves clean and disinfect the coins. One way to do so is:
  - Place all coins in a pot or pan.
  - Liberally add the disinfectant.
  - Add warm water to the pot above the coin level.
  - Do not heat water on the stove. Use warm water from the faucet.
  - Mix the coins around in the pot.
  - Let the coins set in the cleaner for a few minutes.

- Rinse thoroughly, two or three times.
- Remove the coins from the pot and dry.

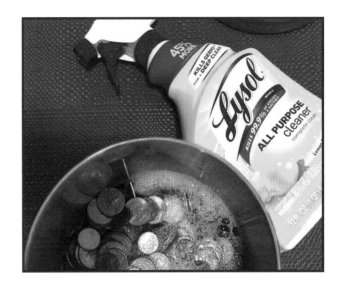

- Place the clean dry coins into the large plastic bowl.
- Clean the Loved One's hands with soap/water and hand sanitizer.
- Place the bowl of coins on the Loved One's lap or a table.
- Let them sift through the coins. Show them how if it is helpful.
- When done, again clean the Loved One's hands with soap/water & hand sanitizer.

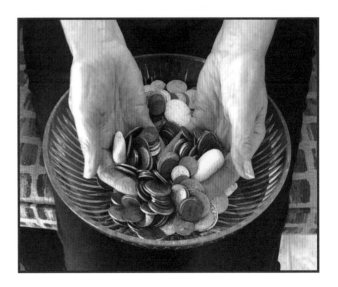

NOTE TO CAREGIVER:

• This is a sensory activity where touch, feel and sound will be different for each Loved One. Different plastic bowls and a different mix of coins will sound and feel different. Experiment to find the combination the Loved One enjoys the most.

SORTING COINS

Stage Appropriate:
Early & Middle

Number of Participants:
1 to 1

This is a fun and productive activity for the Loved One to do. Please remember to disinfect and dry the coins prior to the Loved One handling them.

SAFETY PRECAUTION!

✓ Coins may be a potential choking hazard and may carry harmful germs. Clean the coins thoroughly and always supervise the Loved One during this activity. Following the activity, put all the coins away for safe keeping. Do not heat water on stove, use warm water from the faucet.

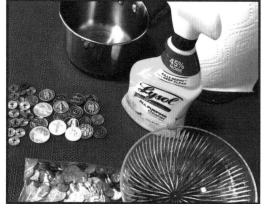

SUPPLIES:

• An assortment of coins

• Clean plastic unbreakable bowls. Four (4) medium size bowls of different colors and one (1) large bowl

• One (1) medium size cooking pot or pan

• A pair of rubber gloves

• Disinfectant, such as Lysol

• Paper or cloth towel

• Hand sanitizer

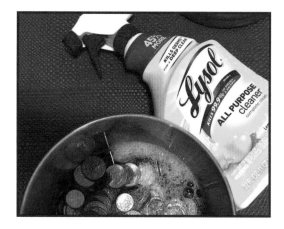

DIRECTIONS:

• Using the pair of rubber gloves, clean and dry the assortment of coins. One way to do so is as follows:

  - Place the assortment of coins in to the cooking pot.

  - Liberally add the disinfectant.

  - Add warm water to the pot above the level of the coins.

  - Mix the coins around in the pot.

  - Let the coins sit in the cleaner for a few minutes.

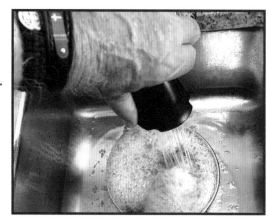

Sorting Coins 2

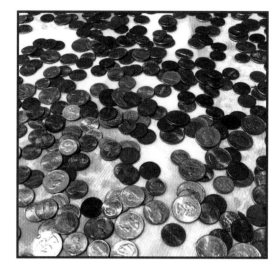

- Pour out the disinfectant & water solution and rinse the coins two (2) or three (3) times.

  - Dry with a towel.

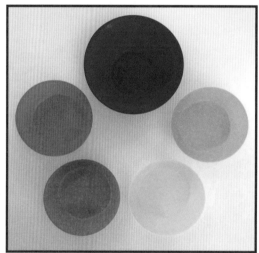

• Place the clean, dry assortment of coins in the large plastic bowl.

• Set out four (4) different colored medium size bowls.

• Show and direct the Loved One how to put like denominations in each bowl.

• If the Loved One is confused by seeing a large assortment of coins, set the large bowl aside and hand a coin, one (1) at a time to the Loved One, to deposit it in a bowl with the same denomination.

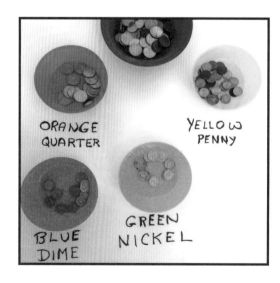

• If necessary you can prompt the Loved One by saying, "put the coin in the red bowl, or blue bowl as the case may be.

• Another prompt could be to write out the color on a card stock and place or tape it to a bowl. Ask that the coin be placed "in the red bowl". (Many Loved Ones retain the ability to read long after they forget "their colors".)

NOTE TO CAREGIVER:

• Another way to clean coins is to make a solution of vinegar and baking soda. Drop a few coins at a time into the solution and watch them fizz. Remove them from the solution, rinse and dry them.

FISH AQUARIUM

Setting up and maintaining

If the caregiver has no prior experience it is recommended that a purchase of a 3 to 5 gallon aquarium is the way to start.

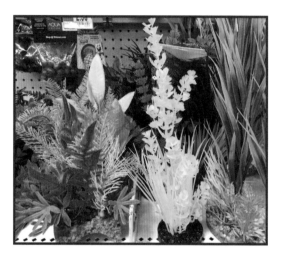

SUPPLIES:

- Aquarium kit which should include:
  - The tank with a cover
  - A filter system with cartridge
  - Light
  - Instructions
- Gravel designated for aquarium use
- Plastic plants
- Air pump if not in kit
- Water conditioner for aquariums
- Heater
- Thermometer
- Fish food

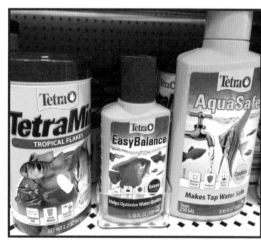

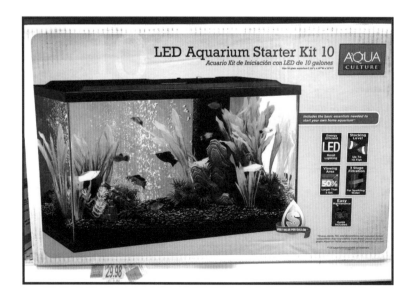

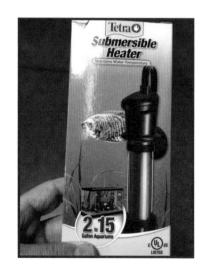

Fish Aquarium 2

DIRECTIONS:

- Select a location for your tank where it is easily visible by the Loved One.

- Wash the inside of the aquarium and all items that will be inside it with warm water.

- Wash and rinse the gravel several times.

- Fill the tank about halfway with room temperature tap water.

- Set up your filter, heater and air pump in the tank.

- Fill the remainder of the tank with water.

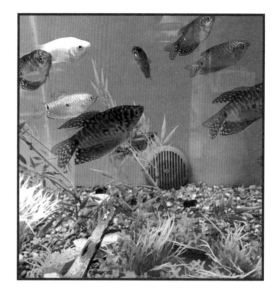

- Add water conditioner according to the instructions.

- Wait 48 hours to give the aquarium time to clear and stabilized. It is normal for the water to be cloudy for a day or so.

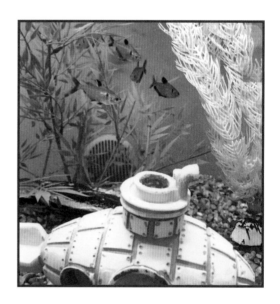

- Now you can go to the pet store and purchase fish.

- Talk to someone who knows all about the different kinds of fish.

- Start with only a few fish. You can always add more later.

- Feed the fish as instructed.

- Enjoy.

NOTE TO CAREGIVER:

- This activity of setting up a tank and caring for the fish is enjoyable for many people. Often just watching the fish is very relaxing.

MEMORY NOTEBOOKS

Keeping Memories Alive

Memory books are not only enjoyable to make, but the Loved One will often carry a book or two with them and flip through the pages repeatedly. Each book should focus on one subject or theme such as cars, pets, family, dolls, old toys. The theme should be one the Loved One most enjoyed in the past.

SUPPLIES:

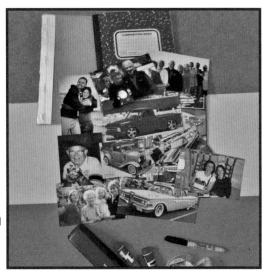

- Small journal notebook.
  (Dollar type stores are a good source)
- Make your own "cereal box notebook"
  (see activity on how to make a cereal box notebook)
- Magazine pictures (Group them into categories or subjects)
- Photos
- Calendar pictures
- Blunt nose scissors, glue, tape, stapler, magic marker or pen

DIRECTIONS:

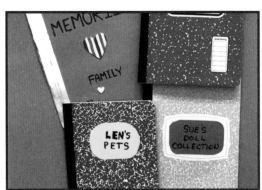

- Choose a single theme.
- From your collection of supplies layout a number of pictures in one category.
- Pick out one photo or picture at a time and show it to the Loved One.
- If the Loved One shows an interest in the picture put it aside to be used.
- Take the pictures or photos the Loved One enjoyed the most and glue, tape or staple them into the notebook.
- Often you can put one larger picture or photo on each page which is easier for the Loved One to focus.
- With a magic marker, in bold print, identify the picture.
- With family pictures print their name.

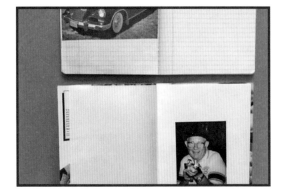

NOTE TO CAREGIVER:

- It is a good idea to put the Loved One's name on the cover of the notebook.

RECYCLED MAGAZINES

Magazines around your house? Here are activities to do with old magazines! Fun, easy, almost free, no right or wrong, and using lots of different skills. We've included many different activities, but it is also fun for mid to late stage Loved Ones to flip through magazines. You will notice a smile when they see something familiar.

SAFETY PRECAUTION!

✓ It is recommended to use children's blunt scissors and glue sticks rather than liquid glue, but either may look like food, so do not leave the Loved One alone with these items.

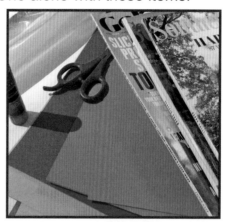

SUPPLIES:

(Used for all the suggested activities)

• Magazines

  - Family Circle and Women's Day are good for: pets, simple foods and large letters

  - Better Homes & Garden is good for garden and home pictures

  - Specialized magazines for golf, fishing, cars, sports, etc. have great pictures

• Children's blunt scissors (fingers for tearing when scissors can't be used)

• Glue sticks

• Paper… construction, card stock, computer paper

• Ziploc type plastic baggies

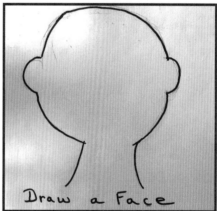

DIRECTIONS:
ACTIVITY NO. 1 MAGAZINE ART

• Decide if you want to make crazy people or crazy animals. Example: Draw the shape of a man's head.

• In a magazine, find and cut out different eyes, ears, body, legs

• Glue onto the man's head, making a very crazy person.

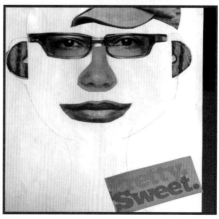

DIRECTIONS:
ACTIVITY NO. 2 WORD HUNTS

Word hunts and making silly sentences are fun ways to keep vocabulary and reading skills alive.

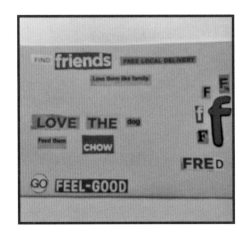

- Cut medium to large size words out of your magazine.
- Put them together to make silly sentences.
- Glue onto paper.
- Read and talk about them together.

NOTE TO CAREGIVER:

- The ability to read is often one of the later remaining skills. If reading and finding words is too difficult, search for letters and make familiar names and words.

DIRECTIONS:
ACTIVITY NO. 3 COLLAGES

- Decide on the theme of your collage… pets, sports, flowers?
- Find and cut out pictures in your magazines that fit your theme. If the Loved One cannot use scissors, tear out the picture and the caregiver can trim them.
- Glue pictures onto a piece of poster board or card stock, or put in a notebook.
- Spread the pictures out on your paper. Simple is best.
- Label the pictures for the Loved One.

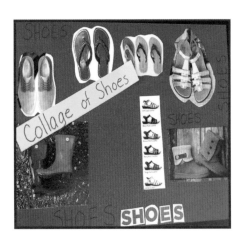

DIRECTIONS:
ACTIVITY NO. 4 STORIES

- Look through magazines and find pictures you will like to use.
- The collection of pictures can be all one theme, very random, or just ones the Loved One wants to cut out.
- After you have the pictures, put them together to tell a story.
- You can also tell a story about just one of the pictures.
- The pictures can remain the same but the stories can vary each time.

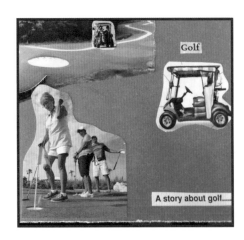

DIRECTIONS:
ACTIVITY NO. 5 "WHAT IS IT?"

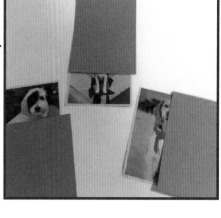

Just for fun guessing game!

• Cut out a fairly large magazine picture of a single item, such as a dog.

• Without the Loved One watching, cover part of the picture with a blank paper.

• Ask the Loved One if he/she can guess what the picture is.

• Show more of the picture if you need to so the Loved One can guess the picture correctly.

• Hints are allowed!

NOTE TO CAREGIVER:

• The pictures you choose will vary depending on the level of the Loved One, from very simple to more detailed. You can ask the Loved One to cover a picture first for you to give him/her the idea.

DIRECTIONS:
ACTIVITY NO. 6 PUZZLES

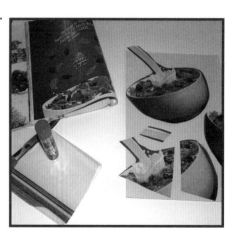

From very simple to difficult, you can make puzzles for the Loved One.

• Cut out pictures, depending on the stage of the Loved One, a simple single object picture for a later stage Loved One, and with more details for earlier stage.

• Glue picture onto cardboard or card stock.

• After pictures dry, cut into pieces. The number of pieces depends on the stage of the Loved One.

• Each puzzle can be put into a Ziploc bag for storage.

DIRECTIONS:
ACTIVITY NO. 7 MATCHING GAME

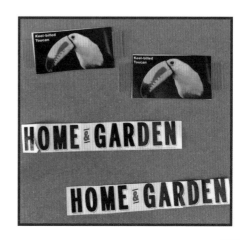

Hooray for duplicate advertisements! This activity can be adapted for each individual with lots of success.

• In your magazines, look for duplicate (2) matching products.

• Repeat this with several different products.

• Place them all together in a pile.

• Pick out one item and ask the Loved One to find the match.

STRING SCAVENGER HUNT

A new version of a scavenger hunt just for the Loved One. He/she will follow the string and find a prize. Sounds fun!!!

SAFETY PRECAUTION!

✓ Be aware of the physical limitations of the Loved One when deciding where to put your string/ribbon. Such as: can they keep their balance and bend down to look under tables or chairs, and is the area free and clear of obstacles that might cause falls?

SUPPLIES:

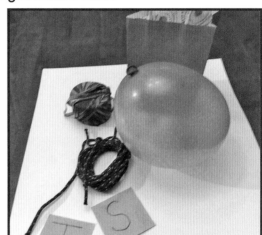

• String or ribbons
  - enough string to wrap around a few chairs, tables, door knobs
• Small prize in a bag or box at the end of the hunt

DIRECTIONS:

• Decide how challenging you can make the course depending on the skill level of the Loved One.
• Decide on the prize for the treasure at the end of the hunt such as:
  - a treat to eat or maybe a small gift.

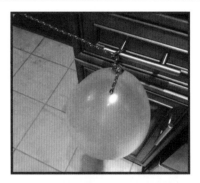

• To begin, tie your string/ribbon around something, such as a door knob or chair. Mark it with something such as a bow, balloon or sign.
• Continue stringing your string/ribbon around furniture in your house.
• Decide where the string ends and the prize will be hidden.
• Tell the Loved One to hold onto the string and follow it until they find the prize.

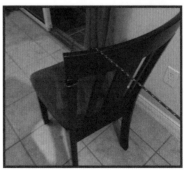

NOTE TO CAREGIVER:

• For early stage Loved Ones, you can place clues for the prize along the string for them to find. You can also place letters of their name along the string, in mixed-up order. They will collect the letters, and at the end, spell their name. For late stage Loved Ones, use a short course and guide them along the string to the prize!

COMMON PHRASES TO COMPLETE

Stage Appropriate:
Early to Middle

Number of Participants:
1 to 3 or more

Completing common phrases is a great way to be successful at language recall. Even wrong answers are fun to hear. You will be surprised at how many of these phrases stay in your memory. For more common phrases: http://www.smart-words.org/quotes-sayings/idioms-meaning.html

SAFETY PRECAUTION!

✓ Be prepared to laugh till it hurts!

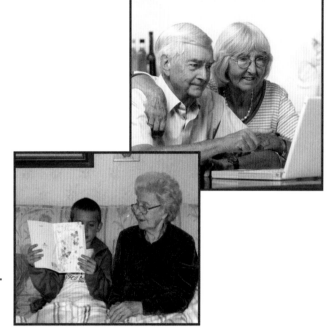

SUPPLIES:

• Access to internet for additional phrases

DIRECTIONS:

• Say the phrase but leave out the underlined word.
• Let the Loved One try to complete the phrase.
• Here are a few to get you started:

"Two wrongs don't make a _right_."

"A penny for your _thoughts_."

"Action speak louder than _words_."

"At the drop of a _hat_."

"Back to the _drawing board_."

"Barking up the wrong _tree_."

"Beat around the _bush_."

"Best thing since sliced _bread_."

"Bite off more than you can _chew_."

"A blessing in _disguise_."

"Can't judge a book by its _cover_."

"Don't cry over spilled _milk_."

"Don't count your chickens before the eggs have _hatched_."

"Don't put all your eggs in one _basket_."

"Kill two birds with one _stone_."

"Let sleeping dogs _lie_."

"Once in a blue _moon_."

"Piece of _cake_."

"See eye to _eye_."

"Speak of the _devil_."

"Straight from the horse's _mouth_."

"Whole nine _yards_."

"Wouldn't be caught _dead_."

"Your guess is as good as _mine_."

"It takes two to _tango_."

"Curiosity killed the _cat_."

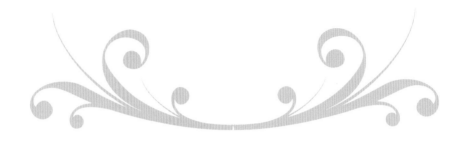

"We must accept finite
disappointment but never
lose infinite hope"

– Dr. Martin Luther King Jr.

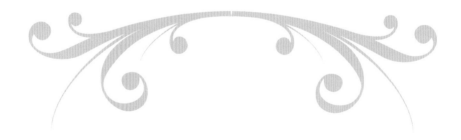

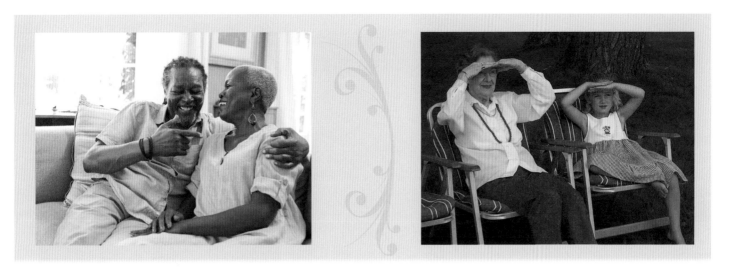

Games And Puzzles

JUST FOR FUN

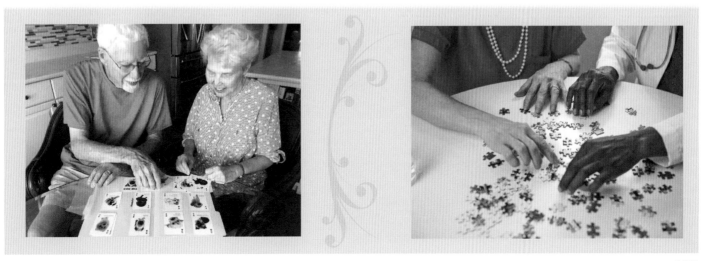

JIGSAW PUZZLES

Fun for Everyone

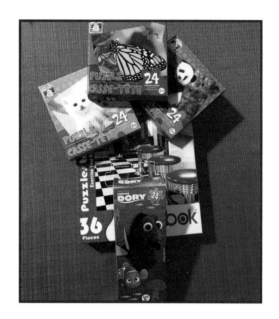

SUPPLIES:

- Store bought jigsaw puzzles
- Solid flat surface
- Comfortable chairs for the caregiver and the Loved One to sit next to each other

DIRECTIONS:

- Puzzles should be appropriate to the abilities of the Loved One and not childish.
- Start with the easiest puzzle you can obtain. Example: a 24 piece puzzle.
- Show the Loved One the completed puzzle.
- Have a picture of the completed puzzle as a guide for the Loved One.
- Take the puzzle apart.
- If the puzzle is too easy, then try a slightly more difficult puzzle. Example: a 36 piece puzzle.
- If the puzzle is too difficult try leaving a few pieces already together before giving it to the Loved One.

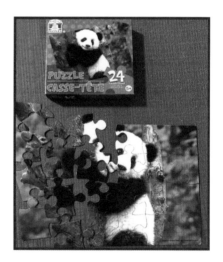

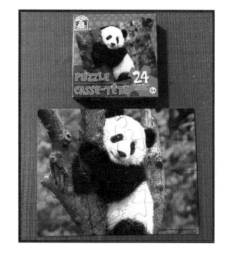

NOTE TO CAREGIVER:

- Dollar type stores are a great source of puzzles.

MAKE A JIGSAW PUZZLE

Specialty puzzles with only a few pieces can be very expensive to purchase. Making your own is inexpensive, relevant and simple. This project is just for the caregiver or someone other than the Loved One to make for the continued use and enjoyment of the Loved One.

DIRECTIONS:
ACTIVITY NO. 1 FOAM BACKED PUZZLE

- Peel and stick foam sheets
- Personal photos, cards or pictures
- Jigsaw template for a 6 to 9 piece puzzle
  (you can go online for samples of templates)
- Scissors
- Scotch tape

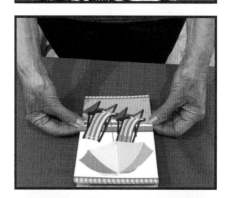

DIRECTIONS:

- Draw your own jigsaw template to the size of the foam sheet you will be using.
- Peel the coating off the sticky side of the foam sheet.
- Select a photo or picture.
- Apply the picture to the sticky side of the foam sheet.
- Turn the foam sheet over.
- Tape the template to this side.
- With scissors cut along the template line.

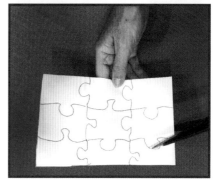

NOTE TO CAREGIVER:
- If you required a puzzle that will get a lot of use consider making one out of plywood.

ACTIVITY NO. 2
PLYWOOD BACKED PUZZLES

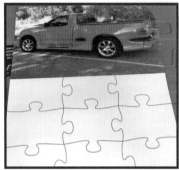

SUPPLIES:

• Aircraft, hobby plywood (thin example 5/32")

• 3M Hi- strength 90 contact adhesive

• Jigsaw puzzle templates

• Photos, cards or pictures

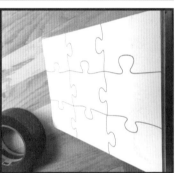

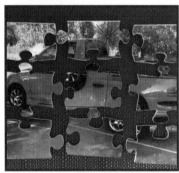

DIRECTIONS:

• Ensure template is the same dimensions as the piece of plywood.

• On one side of the plywood spray the adhesive, following the directions on the container.

• Carefully place the jigsaw template on the sticky surface, press down and let dry.

• Once dried turn the plywood over.

• Spray the adhesive.

• Carefully place the photo, or picture on the sticky surface, press down and let dry.

• Once dried, turn the plywood over and with the jigsaw cut out the pieces of the jigsaw puzzle.

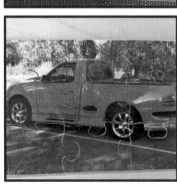

NOTE TO CAREGIVER:

• Photos or pictures can be of familiar items - vehicles, pets, houses, family, items around the house, etc. The more familiar the better.

SHAKE OUT THE "TRUTH"

A fun game that connects people to life events

Stage Appropriate:
Early & Middle

Number of Participants:
1 to 3 or more

Created by Peggy Shelley & Joan Wheeler
Available online at: BestAlzheimersProducts.com

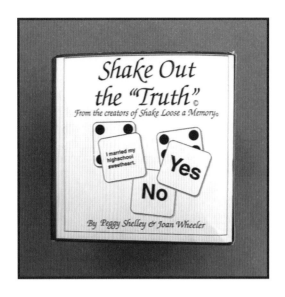

SUPPLIES:

• Shake Out the Truth game

DIRECTIONS:

• Stack cards in order from 1 to 6.

• Distribute Yes/No card to each player.

• Select someone to start the game.

• The first "active" player rolls one die, draws a card matching the die number, reads the event out loud (or someone else reads it for him or her) being careful NOT to give away the truth.

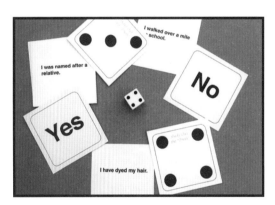

• The remaining player (s) individually show a Yes or NO card depending upon whether they believe the statement is true (Yes) or false (No) about the person reading the card.

• Then the active player gives the truth: Yes or No.

• Encourage everyone to talk about the statement.

• Ways to keep score: Give each player with the right answer a chip or point or item (e.g., piece of candy, penny, etc.). The active player also gets a point for getting the right answer.

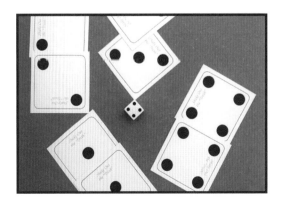

• Repeat this process with each new active player.

NOTE TO CAREGIVER:

• If an active player accidentally gives away the truth before others vote, just have the active player pick another card. Take care to ensure that all players succeed in the game. There are no wrong steps or wrong answers in the game. Have fun!

INDOOR SNOWBALL TOSS

Fun Any Time of Year

Stage Appropriate:
Early, Middle & Late

Number of Participants:
1 to 3 or more

This activity works well for an individual or for groups of any size.

SAFETY PRECAUTION!

✓ Please make sure your artificial snowballs are light and soft so as not to injure anyone or break anything.

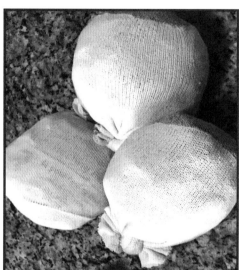

SUPPLIES:

- Decorated (or plain) box or trash can
- Artificial snowballs (available online; brands include Selftek 50 fake snowballs, for $20)
- Or... for homemade snowballs:
  - White tube socks
  - Sheets of paper (cotton balls or fiberfill work too)

DIRECTIONS: HOMEMADE SNOWBALLS

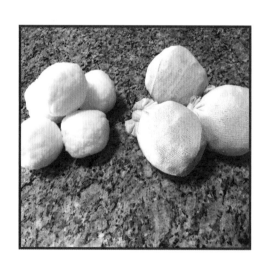

- Stuff crumpled paper (or other material) into the toe end of a sock.
- Shape into the form of a snowball.
- Cut off the sock between the toe and the heel, leaving enough material to either tie or sew the end together.
- Trim excess material.

Indoor Snowball Toss 2

ACTIVITY NO. 1

- Give each Loved One several snowballs.
- One at a time (or however it works out), have players toss their snowballs into a decorated box or trash can.
- Score 1 point for hitting the box.
- Score 2 points for getting a snowball into the container.
- For group play, players might "compete", or they can "always tie", so everyone is a winner!

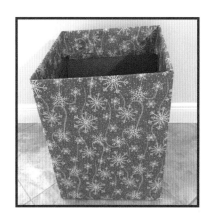

ACTIVITY NO. 2

- Stack small plastic or paper cups into a pyramid. (See cup stacking activity)
- Have Loved Ones throw snowballs at the stack and try to knock down the cups.

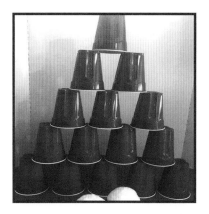

ACTIVITY NO. 3

- Put a target on a wall (e.g., a snowman).
- Hit the snowman with a snowball for a point.

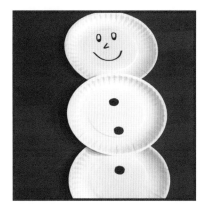

ACTIVITY NO. 4 GROUP

- Choose one or more people to be a "joke teller" or group leader, who will be the friendly target to this game.
- If the joker tells a not-so-funny joke (which is usually the case), then the players will have a great time throwing the soft snowballs at this person.

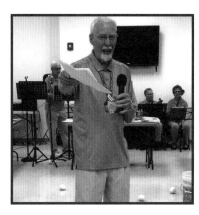

NOTE TO CAREGIVER:

- Late- stage Loved Ones like to hold, squeeze and pat the snowballs.

FILE FOLDER GAMES

Stage Appropriate:
Early & Middle

Number of Participants:
1 to 3 or more

File Folder Games are limitless, almost free, easy to make, easy to use, easy to store, transport and especially fun!

SAFETY PRECAUTION!

✓ Always supervise the Loved One when using scissors, magic markers and glue.

SUPPLIES:

• File Folders, any color
• Ziploc baggies
• Cards to match
• Magazine pictures
• Blunt scissors
• Magic markers
• Glue/glue sticks
• Stickers
• Copy paper

SUPPLIES:
ACTIVITY NO. 1 MATCHING

• Playing cards with different pictures on the cards such as dogs or flowers
• A folder
• Glue
• Ziploc baggie

DIRECTIONS:

• Spread out and glue approximately 10 different card pictures on the inside of the folder.
• Make a deck of matching cards for the Loved One to match to the ones on the file folder.
• Have the Loved One take one card at time and match the card picture to the one in the folder.
• Store the loose cards in a Ziploc baggie.

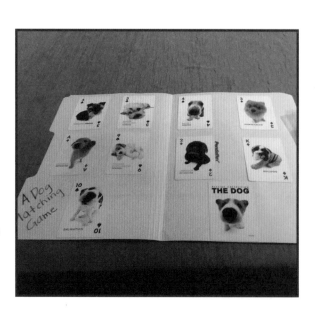

SUPPLIES:
ACTIVITY NO. 2 FAMILY PICTURES MATCH

- Individual photos of family members
- File folder
- Glue
- Magic marker
- Ziploc baggie

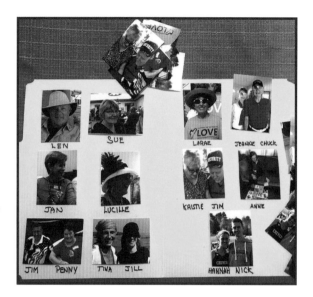

DIRECTIONS:

- Take the individual photos and make 2 prints of each.
- Glue one copy inside the file folder.
- Print the name of the family member under the photo.
- One at a time take the second copy of the photo and hand it to the Loved One to find the match.
- Talk about each photo as you are doing the activity with the Loved One.
- Store the loose photos in a Ziploc bag.

SUPPLIES:
ACTIVITY NO. 3 SHAPES MATCH

- Copy paper
- Scissors
- Magic marker
- Card stock
- File folder
- Ziploc baggie
- Glue

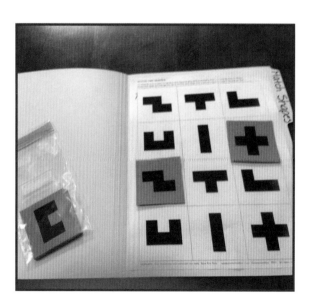

DIRECTIONS:

- Take a piece of copy paper and divide it into 12 sections by drawing the boxes on the paper.
- With the magic marker draw out different shapes.
- Glue the copy paper to the inside cover of the folder.
- Take a piece of card stock and cut into 12 boxes.
- With a magic marker draw the matching shape as seen on the copy paper.
- Store the card stock sections in a baggie.
- To use give one card stock shape to the Loved One and have them find the match.

SUPPLIES:
ACTIVITY NO. 4 MAGAZINE PICTURES MATCH

- Purchase 2 magazines that are identical
- Scissors
- File folder
- Glue
- Ziploc baggie

DIRECTIONS:

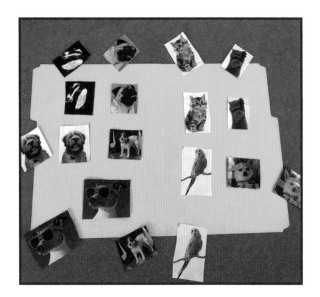

- Locate a picture in the magazine.
- Find the same picture in the other magazine.
- Cut both pictures and set them aside.
- Repeat the process a few times.
- Take one set and glue them to the inside of the folder.
- Have the Loved One take the other set -one at a time- and find the match.
- Store the loose pictures in the baggie.

SUPPLIES:
ACTIVITY NO. 5 COUNTING CARS

- File folder
- Copy paper
- Magic marker with several primary colors
- Glue
- Pencil

DIRECTIONS:

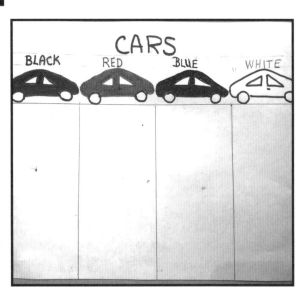

- Line out columns on a piece of copy paper.
- Draw and color 5 cars or so.
- Glue the copy paper of car drawings inside the folder.
- Looking out the window or sitting outside, count and record the cars.

File Folder Games 4

SUPPLIES:
ACTIVITY NO. 6 MAZES

• Magic marker
• Glue
• Folder
• Stickers
• Plain copy paper
• Pencil w/eraser

DIRECTIONS:

• Make two different mazes on copy paper. The way to do so is download "simple mazes" free from the internet.
• Glue a different maze on each inside cover of the file folder.
• Place a sticker at the beginning of the maze and a different one at the end.
• Guide the Loved One to take a pencil and start moving along the maze to the end.
• Erase the results to start over.

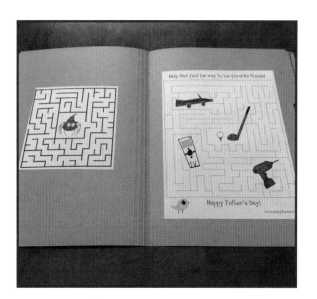

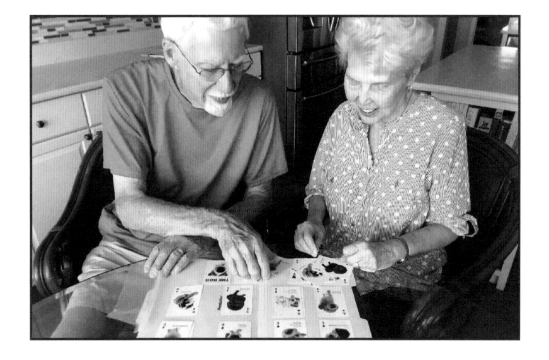

NOTE TO CAREGIVER:

• These activities are not only enjoyable but they can easily be transported to any place you and the Loved One may be.

A TWIST ON "SIMON SAYS"

This is a twist on "Simon Says", making it a great game for exercising your brain and body. "Simon" says: clap your hands 3 times. "Simon" says: kick your right leg 2 times. "Simon" says: touch or point to something blue. Simon's commands can be adapted to each individual's skill level.

SAFETY PRECAUTION!

✓ If balance is an issue with the Loved One, sitting down playing the game is recommended and still a fun activity.

SUPPLIES:

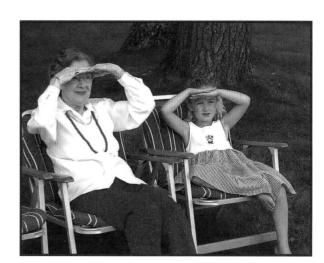

• No supplies are needed
• Play where the Loved One can sit comfortably – living room or kitchen

DIRECTIONS:

• Caregiver will have to demonstrate this activity.

• Explain to the Loved One that "Simon" will give commands and they have to follow.

• Take turns being "Simon" if skill level permits.

• Give commands that exercise the Loved One physically: rub your stomach, pat your head, stomp your feet, etc. Tell how many times to do this action.

• Give commands that exercise the Loved One mentally: count to 15, repeat " I am an awesome person", touch something square, find the letter "R", roar like a lion, etc.

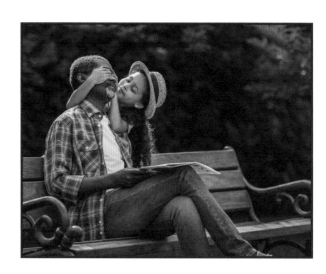

• If the Loved One's skill level permits, try leaving out "Simon says" occasionally... you've tricked them and then it is their turn to be "Simon".

• Use your imagination.

NOTE TO CAREGIVER:

• This is a good activity you can do sitting down, to rest yourself, yet it keeps the Loved One busy. Vary the commands, vary the name "Simon" and make it as silly and fun as possible. This activity can also be used to subtly get the Loved One to do wanted actions, such as brushing their teeth.

SHOE BOX SPORTS

This section is all about indoor sports that you can make and play safely indoors. Using boxes and ping pong balls, a few other supplies and your imagination, you and the Loved One can re-live their sporting days!

SAFETY PRECAUTION!

✓ Markers and paint are often thought of as food items and ping pong balls are small enough to put into the mouth... supervise well.

SUPPLIES:

• Shoe box

• Small diameter dowels, 2 ½" long

• Hole puncher

• 4 or more clothespins

• Markers and/or paint

• Ping pong balls

• Straws

• Duct Tape (optional)

• Cotton balls (optional)

DIRECTIONS:
ACTIVITY NO. 1 FOOSBALL

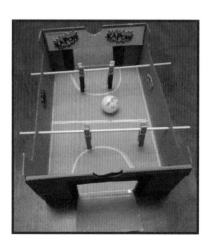

• Color the inside of the box.

• With a marker, add lines similar to a soccer field (Google it).

• Cut an opening at each end of the box for the goals... big enough for a ping pong ball to go into.

• Using a hole puncher, punch 2 holes on both sides of the box to put the dowels through.

• Put faces on clothespins (players).

• Clamp clothespin players onto dowels.

• Using the clothespin players, try to hit the ping pong ball into your goal.

Shoe Box Sports 2

DIRECTIONS:
ACTIVITY NO. 2 AIR SOCCER

(Soccer using straws, ping pong balls and blowing)
- Cut openings at each end of bottom box large enough for a ping pong ball to go through.
- Decorate box with paint/markers/stickers to resemble a soccer field.
- Using a straw, blow the ping pong ball or cotton ball through the hole = goal.
- Keep score and have prizes if desired.

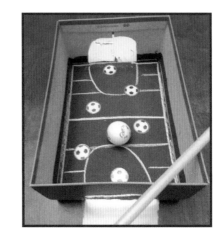

DIRECTIONS:
ACTIVITY NO. 3 SHOE BOX BASKETBALL

- Turn the top of the shoe box upside down. This will be your basketball court.
- Decorate your court.
- Cut a hole (hoop) into each end of the top of the shoe box so the ball can drop to the bottom of the box.
- Set the top box on the bottom one and secure with tape.
- Put the ping pong ball on the basketball court and the Loved One will tip the box enough to get the ball into the hoops. This is a basket and 2 points!

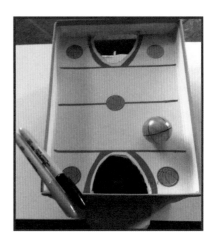

DIRECTIONS:
ACTIVITY NO. 4 INDOOR GOLF

You will need a putter and a golf ball.
- Cut top off box
- Turn the box upside down and cut 2 openings on the side of the box for the putting holes. Make sure the holes are large enough for the balls to fit through.
- Paint and decorate.
- Use duct tape to mark the fairway.
- Putt the balls through the holes.

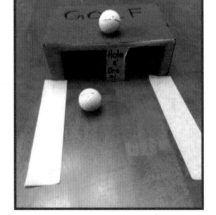

NOTE TO CAREGIVER:
- For the "tennis" pro, blow up a balloon and use a flyswatter to hit the balloon back and forth. For this activity make sure the Loved One is sitting down in a secure, sturdy chair.

CARD GAMES

Fun for Everyone

Card games are for everyone! There are card games for all levels of play. Go Fish, Crazy Eight, Memory Game and War! Old Maid, UNO and Photo Cards! Games can be played using the original rules, or with very simple adaptations! There are so many benefits to playing cards: fine motor skills and eye-hand coordination improve, exercising your mind, and interaction with each other. Remember to have fun! Here are a few ideas.

SUPPLIES:

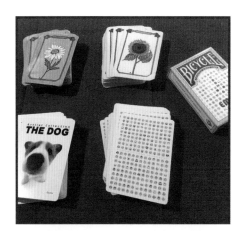

- 4+ decks of cards with a variety of designs on the back
- Optional: Poster board, cardboard or the inside blank side of cereal boxes
- Glue stick

DIRECTIONS:
ACTIVITY NO. 1 MATCHING PICTURES

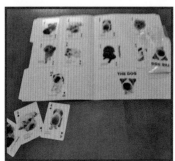

- Glue 6 or more cards, facing up, onto the poster board. The number you use depends on the skill level of the Loved One.
- Alternate using red/black cards to limit confusion.
- Gluing is optional. You can just lay them down.
- Using cards from the 2nd deck, the Loved One will match the cards that are laid down.
- The number of cards you give from the 2nd deck will be determined by the skill of the Loved One.

DIRECTIONS:
ACTIVITY NO. 2 MATCHING NUMBERS

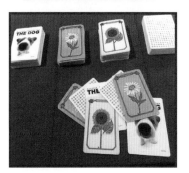

- Match and sort the backs of several different decks of cards.
- Match and sort using the numbers and symbols.
- Match and sort using red and black suits.
- UNO cards are great for matching.
- You can also print doubles of family pictures, glued to old cards, and play a family matching game.

DIRECTIONS:
ACTIVITY NO. 3 UNO

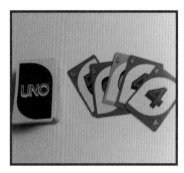

- Play by the rules.
- Play with your own rules some ways include:
  - Sort by color.
  - Sort by number.
  - Sort by color and number.
  - The caregiver can reduce the size of the deck and play a simplified game with the original rules.

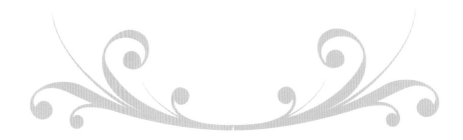

**Come to me, all you who
are weary and burdened
and I will give you rest**

Matthew 11:28

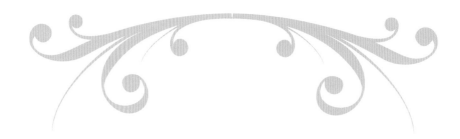

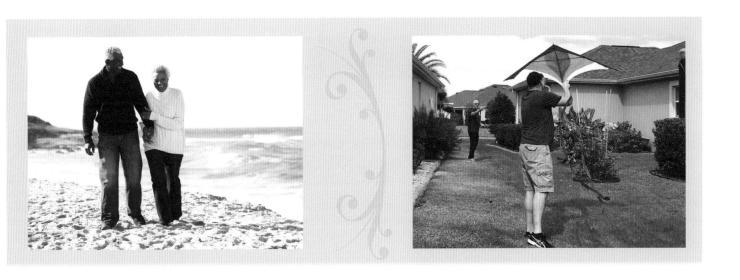

*T*hings *T*o *D*o *O*utside

THERE IS BEAUTY AND JOY THAT SURROUNDS US.
STEP OUTSIDE AND SHARE A MOMENT,
QUIETLY WITH THE LOVED ONE.

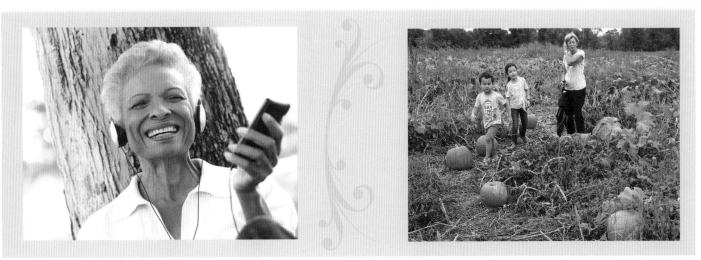

EARLY MEMORIES

Early memories may stay with the Loved One the longest. This activity can bring you together as you and the Loved One look at early toys, appliances, games, etc.

SUPPLIES:

• Cell phone with camera

• Computer or tablet device like an iPad

• Antique consignment shop or large antique store

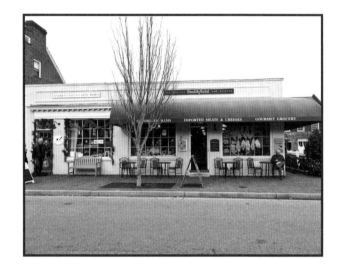

DIRECTIONS:

• The caregiver should go to a local antique consignment shop or store.

• Take pictures of items the Loved One might have used or seen in their early years.

• When at home transfer the pictures to your computer or tablet.

• Sitting beside the Loved One, look at each picture and talk about it.

(Sample pictures on the next page)

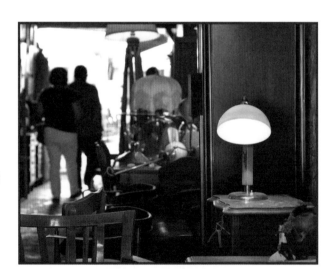

NOTE TO CAREGIVER:

• It is a good idea to ask the shop proprietor for permission to photograph the items. When taking photos, concentrate on trying to take pictures of individual items.

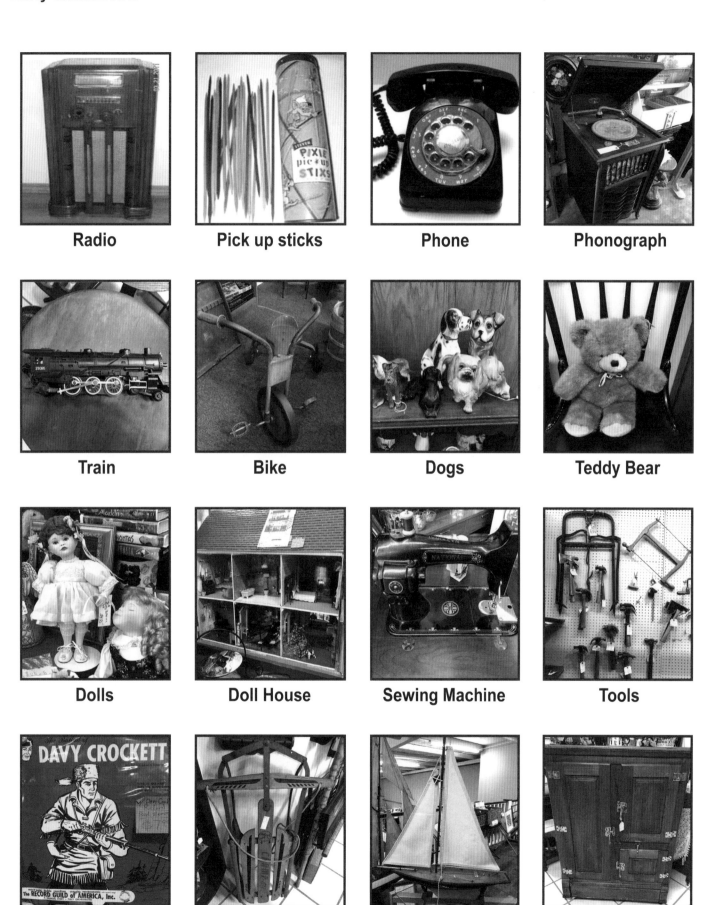

Radio	Pick up sticks	Phone	Phonograph
Train	Bike	Dogs	Teddy Bear
Dolls	Doll House	Sewing Machine	Tools
Davy Crockett	Sled	Sailboat	Ice Box

NATURE SIGHTSEEING

Stage Appropriate:
Early, Middle & Some Late

Number of Participants:
1 or more

God's Pallet

There are many ways to observe nature in all its beauty. You can simply sit out on a porch, in your yard, driveway or expand geographically out from there. Remember in a natural, quiet setting, concentrate on all the senses: sight, smell, hearing, taste & touch.

SUPPLIES:

• None necessary

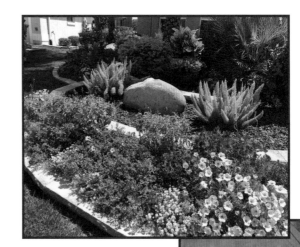

DIRECTIONS:

• Start simply in your yard or driveway. Walk or sit and look around.

• Ask the Loved One if he/she sees or hears what you see or hear.

• Grab a hand full of dirty grass, pick a flower or leaf.

• Share what you see, hear and smell with the Loved One.

• Make the Loved One aware of how the sun, wind, air temperature is sensed.

• Expand your sightseeing opportunities to consider beaches, lakes, city parks, zoos, mountains and a place to view beautiful sunsets.If you are limited with mobility much can be viewed while sitting in a car.

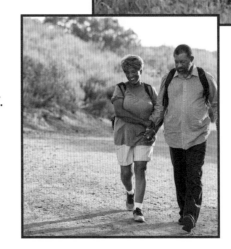

Nature Sight Seeing 2

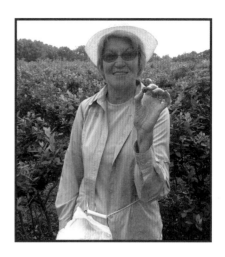

- There are other ways to see nature including:
  - Gardening or yard work.
  - Watching a couple of fish in a small fish bowl.
  - Feeding ducks and birds.
  - Going fruit picking for apples and berries.
  - Playing in snow.

NOTE TO CAREGIVER:

- There are many positive health benefits to being outside communing with nature. Some benefits are increased absorption of vitamin D, reduction of stress and hypertension and reduction of blood pressure. When we experience the power of nature we find it soothing and we naturally feel better.

Additional ideas if you are unable to spend much outside time include: Thumbing through nature magazines and calendars, viewing YouTube footage on nature such as: Peaceful Relaxing Music and Calming Nature Sounds, Bird Song Sounds, and Nature Sounds of the Forest.

A personal note: During one of the last days of my mother's life we sat quietly out in her driveway. We heard a bird sing. My mother asked, What is that? Listen, I answered, the bird is saying it's name – Chickadee – dee - dee – Chickadee – dee- dee. With a big beautiful smile my mother repeated Chickadee – dee – dee several times. Each time the bird called back Chickadee – dee- dee; this was one of the most peaceful times in our lives.

There is no limit to the way God can communicate with you.

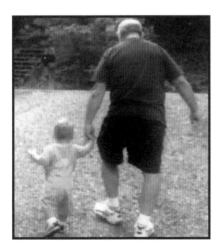
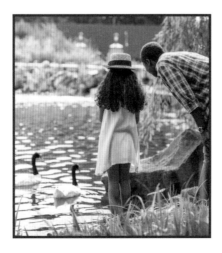
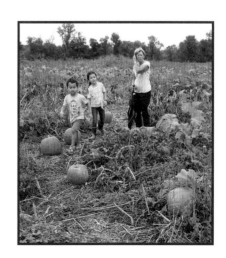

GO FLY A KITE

Up, Up and Away

Flying a kite today is a lot easier than it was even a few years ago.
There is no running or wild erratic motions necessary to fly a kite well.

SAFETY PRECAUTION!

✓ For the Loved One as well as the caregiver absolutely <u>no running</u> or <u>even walking</u>, especially walking backwards. No activity should involve walking backward. You just stand or sit. Do not fly a kite near power lines and trees.

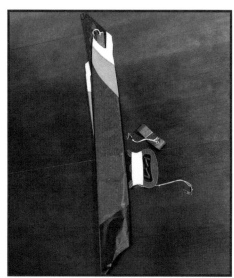

SUPPLIES:

• Purchase a kite. Not just any kite. It is recommended you go to a hobby store or online and search for a "single line" kite for beginners (adult and children). One very reputable, dependable, easy to assemble and fly kite is a "Single String Delta easy- flier kite". The kites today come complete with everything needed.

• Homemade kites and "Five and Dime" novelty toy kites are not as easy to fly as one of the newer, well-engineered brand name kites of today.

• An assistant to help the caregiver and the Loved One fly the kite.

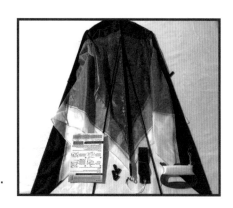

DIRECTIONS:

• Read and follow the assembly instructions. For these beginner kites the instructions are 3 steps or less.

• Attach your kite flying line securely.

• Find an open space to fly your kite. In the street, near power lines and trees <u>is not</u> acceptable. It is unsafe.

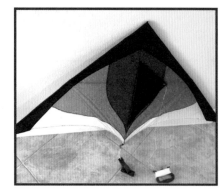

Go Fly A Kite 2

- To fly the kite into the air the caregiver should hold the kite line while an assistant holds the kite about 45 to 55 feet away.

- The kite line should be held tightly.

- The wind should be blowing directly on the back of the caregiver holding the kite.

- When the caregiver is ready, the assistant should be signaled to let go of the kite line.

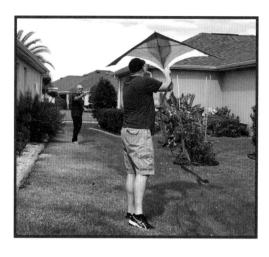

- <u>NO ONE – NO ONE IS TO RUN OR WALK BACKWARDS</u>. Running will not help the kite fly. Actually, running will work against the kite flying and RUNNING WHILE TRYING TO FLY A KITE IS DANGEROUS AND NOT TO BE DONE. THE KITE WILL FLY WHEN THE ASSISTANT LETS IT GO IN A STEADY BREEZE.

- To assist the kite to climb, the caregiver can "pump" the kite line or just pull in a little line and then lift it up. No walking backwards.

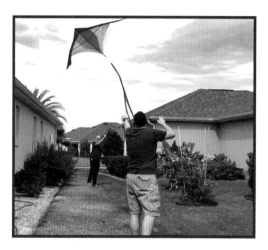

- Once in the air the kite will stay flying until the wind stops or it is reeled in.

- At this point give the kite line to the Loved One who will be flying the kite.

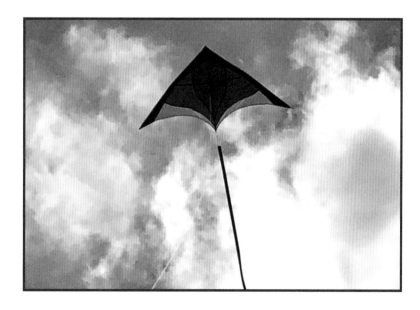

NOTE TO CAREGIVER:

- If the wind is steady the kite will fly easily. Be safe, be patient and enjoy your time with nature, the beauty of the day, and the Loved One. This moment is a joyful gift.

WALK ON THE BEACH

This is one of many types of nature outings that are healthy and enjoyable. Other destinations extend from your own backyard to paths through the woods, parks, etc. !

SAFETY PRECAUTION!

✓ Be very careful to evaluate the health, ability, energy, capacity and safety of the Loved One. Even just going out in the yard requires prior planning. Prior planning includes elements of transportation, food, water, the continuous needs of the Loved One and your own personal limitations and ability to take a Loved One outside. Taking along neighbors and friends is always to be considered.

SUPPLIES:

- Cellphone
- Proper clothing, possibly an extra coat
- Proper footwear
- Any assistive device such as: cane, walker or wheelchair
- People or a person to assist
- Sunglasses
- Water and possibly a snack
- Head cover such as: cap or hat
- A bag to hold found "treasures"
- A pre- prepared plan

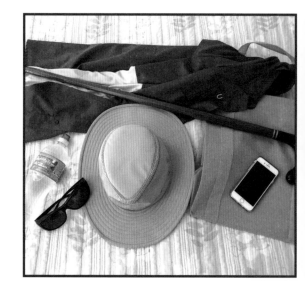

DIRECTIONS:

- As you prepare for your nature walk even though you have a plan, make a final assessment of your ability, the Loved One's current condition and the weather. If all is not perfect just put it off for another day.

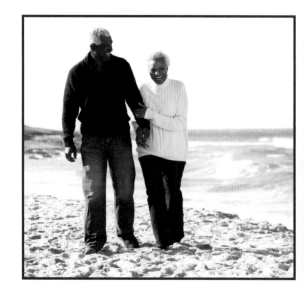

Walk On The Beach 2

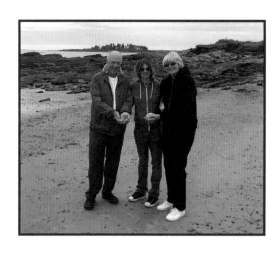

- When at the beach you can often park in a place where you can sit and hear people talking and watch what they are doing.

  - Notice the action of the waves, the birds, clouds and other features of nature.

- If able you can venture out onto the beach. Searching for treasures is great. Sand, stones and shells are great treasures to be saved.

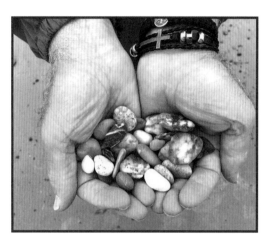

- Take time to sit in the sand and build a sand castle.

- Check with the Loved One often to see how they are doing. Do not go too far from the car. Keep it in sight. No need to walk far.

- This activity is for fresh air, seeing nature at its best and sharing. It is not for the purpose of "getting a workout" or exercise.

- Use your beach chairs, sit and enjoy.

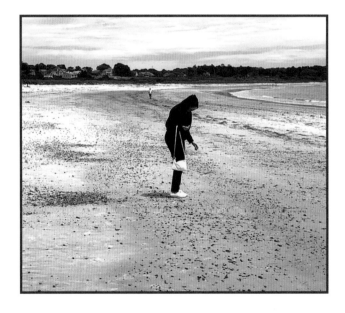

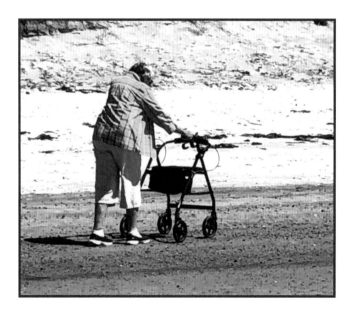

NOTE TO CAREGIVER:

- Enjoy this activity with the Loved One. It may turn out to be one of the most memorable ever. I will always have a warm memory of my Loved One carrying her pocket book while "walking" and enjoying the day.

OUR TRIPS...OUR STORIES

Fun for Everyone

Stage Appropriate:
Early to Middle

Number of Participants:
1 to 1

A fun way to reminisce together! Telling stories about your trips, looking at pictures and making your stops on the map.

SAFETY PRECAUTION!

✓ Provide supervision when markers are being used.

SUPPLIES:

• Map of US and/or the World
• Notebook/pen
• Photos
• Markers

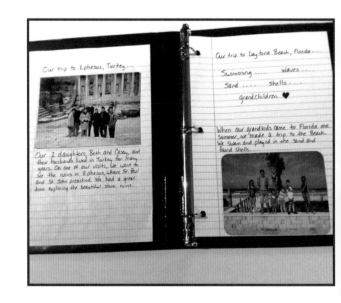

DIRECTIONS:

• Pick a place you have visited together.
• Find it on the map and mark it.
• Write down memories you have of this trip.
• Include pictures if you have any (Pictures might help remind the Loved One of the trip).
• This can be an ongoing together activity.

NOTE TO CAREGIVER:

• This can also be done with places you have lived together.

VEHICLES AND MORE...

Pull up a chair, sit on a bench and become vehicle, people and animal watchers!

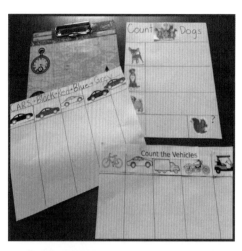

SAFETY PRECAUTION!

✓ Watch out for traffic!

SUPPLIES:

• Clipboard

• Pencil/pen

• Paper

• Drawings of vehicles, pictures of cars, dogs, birds, etc.

• File Folders

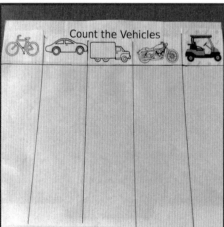

DIRECTIONS:

• Download vehicle/animal/people pictures from the internet or draw your own.

• Make a simple chart to track numbers of vehicles/animals/walkers you see.

• You can also draw and color different cars and see how many of each color you see.

• Store and carry these games on a clipboard. Take them anywhere you go.

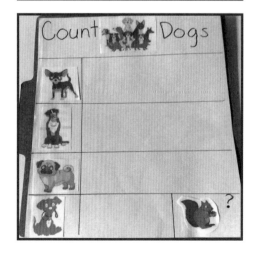

NOTE TO CAREGIVER:

• It's a lot of fun to create your own clipboard together to be used for drawing, writing, or holding a paper game (see the Activity Decorating Clipboards).

SEED PLANTING

Planting and taking care of the plants and watching them grow is a great activity. These plants are suggested for inside the house or porch so the Loved One can "keep an eye" on their growth.

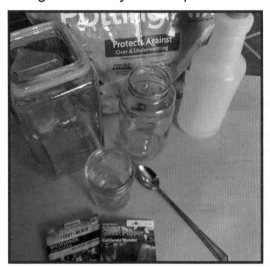

SAFETY PRECAUTION!

✓ Seeds and dirt might look tempting to eat! Always be with the Loved One during this project!

SUPPLIES:

- Dirt (You can use potting soil, but plain dirt is good too)
- Bean seeds, marigold seeds, or grass seeds
- Clear plastic cup or glass jar
- Spoon
- Water

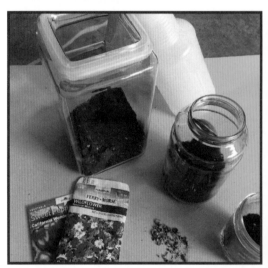

DIRECTIONS:

- Pick out the plants you would like to grow.
- Put dirt into cup or jar.
- With the handle of the spoon, poke some holes in dirt.
- Drop in seeds.
- Cover with dirt.
- Water.
- Watch your plant grow fast!

NOTE TO CAREGIVER:

- If you choose to use grass seeds, a fun thing to do is draw a face with permanent marker onto the plastic cup. Grass will grow fast and will look like green hair sticking up! Most of the other plants can be transferred outside after they reach 4" tall.

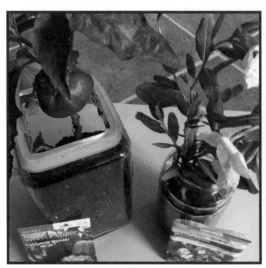

CELL PHONE WALK

SAFETY PRECAUTION!

✓ Do not wander too far.

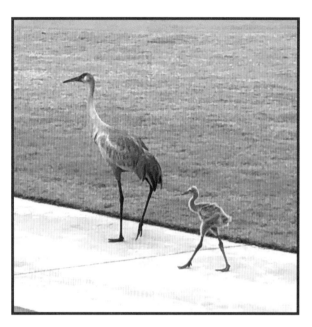

SUPPLIES:

- A nice day outside
- Cell phone
- An assistive device as necessary, such as a walking stick, cane, wheelchair, etc.

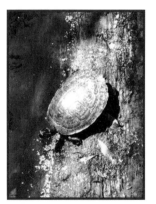
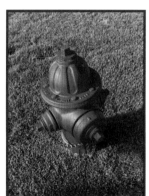

DIRECTIONS:

- "Mosey" along slowly- very slowly, walk, amble or ride along. While doing so, take pictures with a cell phone and talk about what you see.

- As you move forward, focus on the things you sense around you.

- Look and point out flowers, clouds, birds, trees, houses, etc. Take time to study each one.

- Have the Loved One point to items of interest too.

- Take a cell phone picture of the things you talked about. Try to isolate each object from other distractions as much as possible.

- When you return, review and talk about the pictures you saw on your walk.

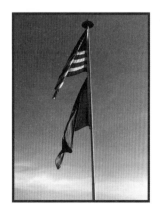
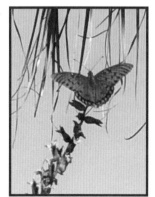

NOTE TO CAREGIVER:

- If the Loved One cannot journey outside, a "cell phone" walk inside the house works also.

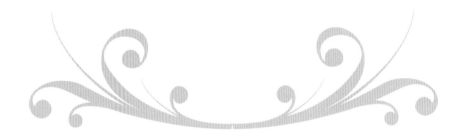

"Optimism is the faith
that leads to achievement"

– Helen Keller

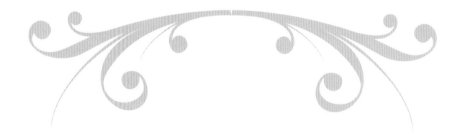

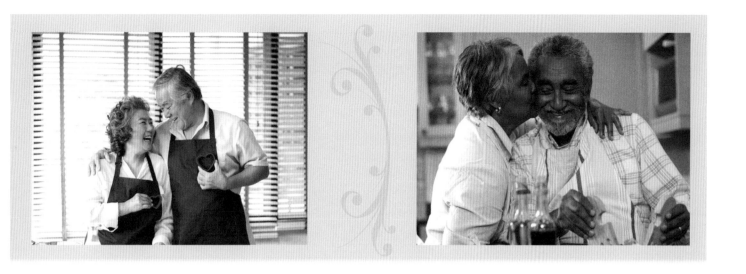

*F*ood *F*or *F*oodies

FUN TO DO
ENJOYABLE TO EAT

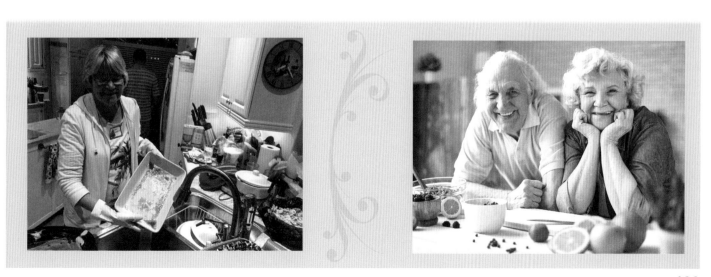

ZIPLOC BAG OMELET(S)

Fun And Delicious

Most people agree, once you prepare an omelet in this way you will do it often. It is very easy and the omelet is delicious.

SAFETY PRECAUTION!

✓ This activity involves boiling water and hot contents in a Ziploc bag. Only the caregiver is to perform this part of the activity, regardless of the capabilities of the Loved One.
All chopped vegetables should be prepared by the caregiver.

SUPPLIES:

• Quart size Ziploc bag

• Two eggs per person

• Variety of chosen ingredients such as:
- diced onions   - bacon
- shredded cheese   - sliced mushrooms
- chopped ham   - chopped sausage

• A two quart pot will accomodate 2 omelets.

• Tongs

• Pot holder or oven mitts

• Seasoning (salt, pepper or other)

• Scissors

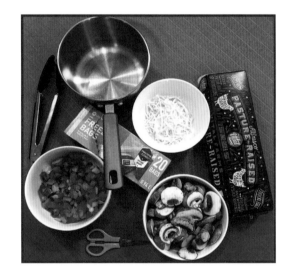

DIRECTIONS:

• Fill pot half way with water.

• Crack open an egg and empty the contents into one Ziploc bag. Repeat so that there are two eggs in each Ziploc bag to serve each person.

• Seal the bag and have the Loved One mush the eggs together in the bag.

• The caregiver should open the bag and the Loved One select and add their ingredients.

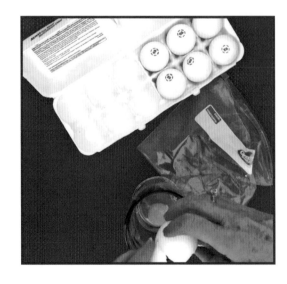

Ziploc Bag Omelet(s) 2

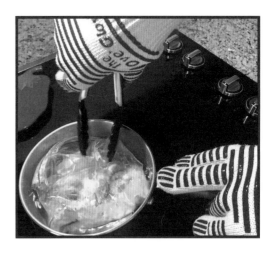

• Close the bag again and have the Loved One mush together the contents. Make sure it's well sealed.

• Place the pot of water on the stove and bring it to a boil. (This is to be done by the caregiver only).

• Using the tongs place the bag(s) carefully into the boiling water.

• Boil for seven (7) minutes .

• Turn off the stove.

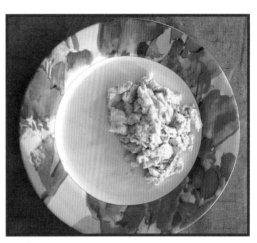

• With the tongs, remove the Ziploc bags from the pot and place on a plate. (Safely keep this step of the activity away from the Loved One).

• Hold the bag with the tongs or oven mitt, and with the scissors cut open the bag. (Caution: bag and contents are very hot).

• Hold the corners of the bottom of the bag using the oven mitt and slide the omelet onto a plate.

• Season as desired.

• Serve toast with butter, jelly or cinnamon sugar if desired.

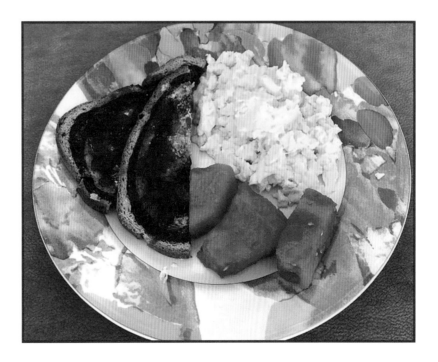

NOTE TO CAREGIVER:

• Sometimes the Loved One's participation may be limited by safety precautions, however, they may enjoy watching the other part of the process from a safe distance and really enjoy the mushing process and toast preparation.

MAKE AND DECORATE CUPCAKES

Cupcakes or muffins are easy to make and fun to decorate and as always the goal is to have an enjoyable activity together regardless of what the end process may look like.

SAFETY PRECAUTION!

✓ All parts of this activity around a hot oven must be performed by the caregiver with the Loved One at a safe distance.

SUPPLIES:

- Cake mix
- Large mixing bowl
- Eggs
- Water
- Spatula
- Frosting
- Candy sprinkles
- Various small candy
- Oven mitts
- Muffin pan
- Cupcake liners
- Butter
- Mixer
- Spoons
- Decorating kit
- Candy eyes
- Pretzels

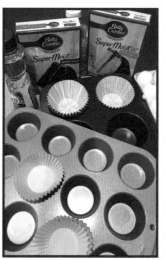
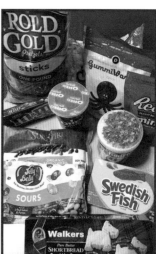

DIRECTIONS:

- Following the directions on the cake mix box:
  - Combine the cake mix, butter, water, in a large bowl and mix.
  - Line the muffin pan with the cupcake liners.
  - Fill each liner with two thirds 2/3 of the mix.
  - Bake for twenty (20) minutes on 350 degrees.
  - Remove from oven with oven mitts.
  - Cool the cupcake completely before decorating.
- Spread the frosting onto the top of the cupcake with the spatula.
- Decorate.

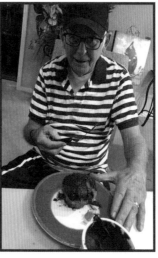
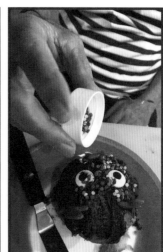

Make And Decorate Cupcakes 2

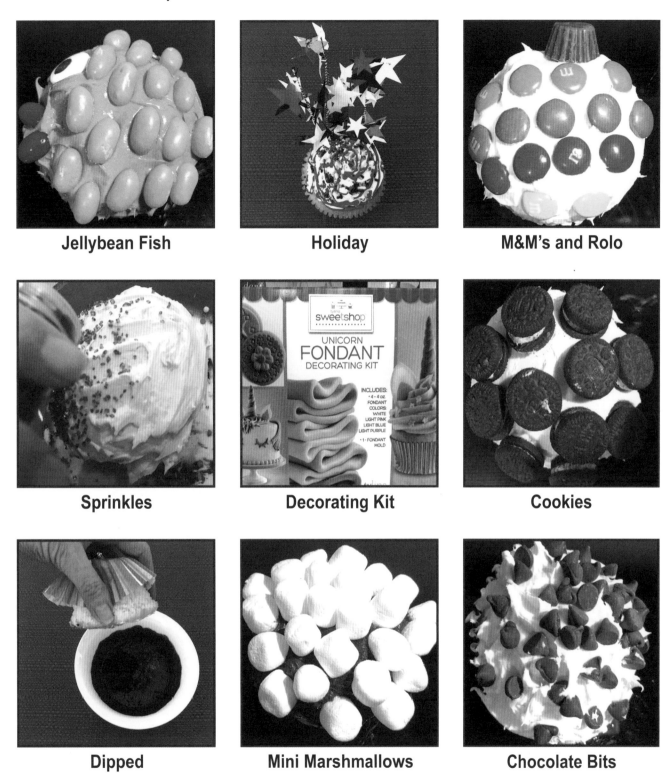

Jellybean Fish

Holiday

M&M's and Rolo

Sprinkles

Decorating Kit

Cookies

Dipped

Mini Marshmallows

Chocolate Bits

NOTE TO CAREGIVER:

• Calories can be reduced by using half as much butter called for in the recipe or substituting ½ cup of butter with ¼ cup of apple sauce. Also if the Loved One cannot spread the frosting with the spatula melt frosting in a microwave safe bowl in the microwave. Remove with oven mitts, place on safe surface and dip the top of the cupcake in the melted frosting.

COFFEE CUP MICROWAVE SCRAMBLED EGGS

This activity is so simple to do, and the eggs are so fluffy and enjoyable you may never scramble eggs any other way in the future.

SAFETY PRECAUTION!

✓ Make sure the cup is microwave safe. When removing the cup (which must be microwave safe) from the microwave the cup and contents will be very hot. Let it cool or remove the eggs from the cup on a plate before eating.

SUPPLIES:

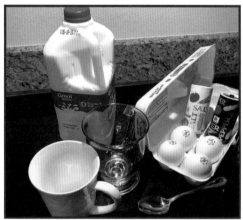

- Two (2) eggs per person and per cup
- Milk
- Spice as desired such as salt, pepper and cinnamon
- Oven mitts
- One (1) large microwave safe coffee cup
- Spoon

DIRECTIONS:

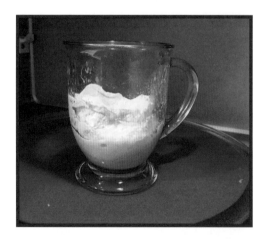

- Take two (2) eggs, break and empty the contents into the coffee cup.
- Add a touch of milk.
- Whip the milk and eggs until blended.
- Place into the microwave and heat on high for one (1) minute.
- Remove the cup from the microwave with oven mitts.
- Stir the contents of the cup until blended.
- Place the cup back into the microwave and heat on high for fifteen(15) seconds.
- Remove the cup with oven mitts and scoop the contents into a plate.
- Season as desired.

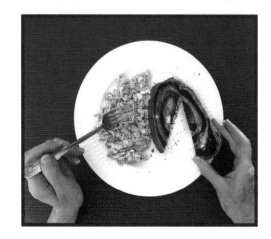

NOTE TO CAREGIVER:

- ENJOY!

FIXING FRESH VEGGIES

This activity helps to keep the Loved One busy, productive, helpful and healthy.

SAFETY PRECAUTION!

✓ The caregiver should pre-cut all the veggies before doing this activity. Alternatively the caregiver could select pre-cut and pre-prepared veggies.

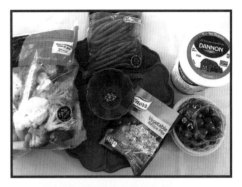

SUPPLIES:

- Pre-cut or fresh veggies of your choice
- Colander
- Paper towels
- Large unbreakable salad bowl
- Large unbreakable serving plate
- Dip mix
- Cottage cheese
- Cream cheese

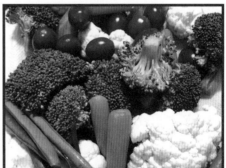

DIRECTIONS:

- Place veggies in a colander.
- Rinse veggies and towel dry.
- If needed pull apart broccoli and cauliflower florets.
- Optional
  - Cut celery sticks to size
  - Peel carrots
  - Cut tomatoes
- Arrange on a large serving plate as a veggie platter.

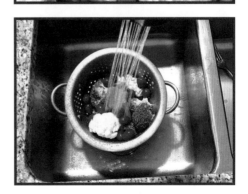

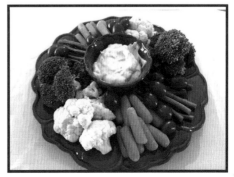

ENGLISH MUFFINS PIZZA

A Simple and Yummy Activity

This is a great skill building activity. The Loved One will feel helpful and proud of their pizza.

SAFETY PRECAUTION!

✓ The caregiver should pre-cut all the toppings before doing the activity.

SUPPLIES:

- English muffins
- Pizza sauce
- Shredded mozzarella cheese
- Assortment of toppings: peppers, onion, mushrooms, ham, pepperoni, pineapple, etc.
- Oven cookie sheet

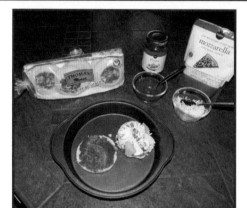

DIRECTIONS:

- Wash fresh toppings.
- Place the English Muffin halves onto a cookie sheet.
- Spoon pizza sauce onto the muffin halves.
- Add the toppings and mozzarella cheese.
- Bake for 10 minutes or until cheese is melted. (320°)
- Cool slightly, eat and enjoy!

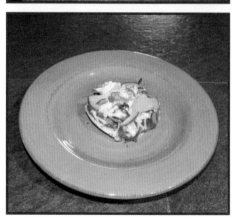

NOTE TO CAREGIVER:

- Be sure to take pictures of this activity and talk about it often. You can also make a fruit pizza, using flavored yogurt and slices of fruit on a hot toasted muffin.

CRACKERS AND .....?

This activity is so simple, so fun, so yummy… creating toppings for crackers. Putting different toppings together, layering them, eating cold, or microwaving them are all possibilities. The Loved One can use many different skills making these and at the same time feel helpful and successful.

SAFETY PRECAUTION!

✓ Watch for food items that might cause choking. The caregiver should pre-cut the ingredients to be used.

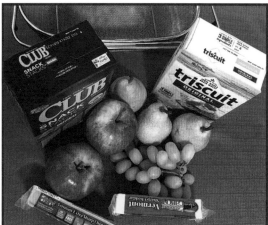

SUPPLIES:

- Any shape cracker
- Peanut butter
- Cheese
- Strawberries, apples
- Chocolate such as Nutella
- Lunch meat
- Sliced veggies
- Cream cheese
- Plastic knife

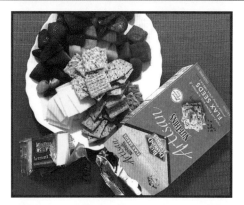

DIRECTIONS:

- Show the Loved One a sample cracker with toppings and explain you are going to make fancy crackers today.
- Decide with the Loved One what toppings to use on your crackers.
- Create using any combinations.
- If melting cheese… microwave for seconds.
- Sample many different combinations and decide which is your favorite.

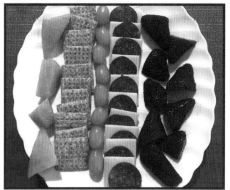

NOTE TO CAREGIVER:

- Be sure to take pictures of the Loved One making these crackers. This is a good activity for Your Loved One to feel helpful.

IT'S PARTY TIME WITH CHEX MIX AND MORE!

This is a fun and yummy snack for you and the Loved One to make together. The options of ingredient are up to you and will be determined by what the Loved One can safely eat and enjoy.

SAFETY PRECAUTION!

✓ When deciding on the ingredients, make sure the Loved One will not choke on peanuts and popcorn. This is still a yummy treat without those ingredients.

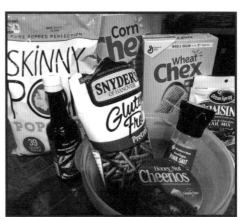

SUPPLIES:

- Chex Mix
- Cheerios
- Pretzels
- Popcorn (Kettle Korn!)
- Peanuts (Depends on your Loved One)
- Your ideas
- Mixing bowls
- Storage bags

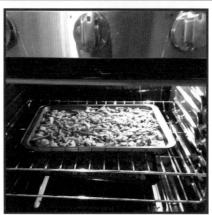

DIRECTIONS:

- Let the Loved One really help choose the ingredients (but you have the initial choice).
- Add your ingredients and stir
- Bake at 325° for 1 hour. Mix every 15 minutes.
- Eat and enjoy!

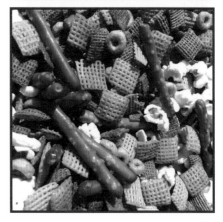

NOTE TO CAREGIVER:

- This is such a fun and easy snack to make and the Loved One will feel useful. Package the snack and it will last for a while. Save your cereal boxes to make games and books.

IT'S NOT JUST PUDDING!

It's a together project. It's a yummy delicious project.

SAFETY PRECAUTION!

✓ The caregiver should pre-cut the ingredients to be used.

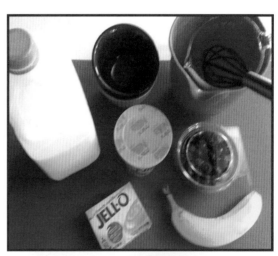

SUPPLIES:

• Instant Pudding
• Milk
• Toppings such as:
  - strawberries
  - blueberries
  - bananas
  - granola
  - broken pretzels
  - whipped cream
• Wisk
• Spoons

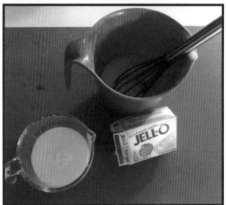

DIRECTIONS:

• Mix pudding according to directions on the box.
• Talk about the different toppings and pick what you would like to use.
• Layer toppings and pudding or just put toppings on top.
• Chill for a short time.

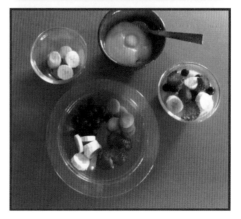

NOTE TO CAREGIVER:

• By using clear bowls or cups, you can see all the layered toppings.

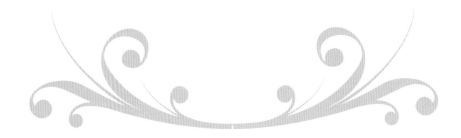

**"Most of us have more courage
than we ever dreamed
we possessed"**

– Dale Carnegie

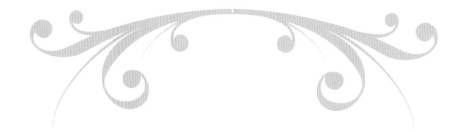

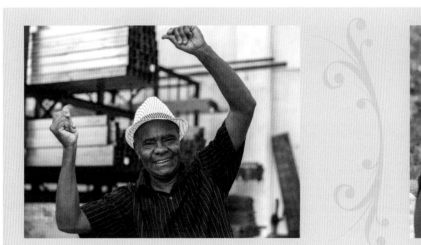
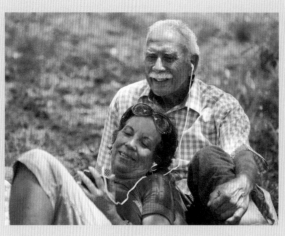

*M*usic *T*o *M*y *E*ars

MUSIC CAN:
REDUCE ANXIETY AND DEPRESSION
REDUCE AGITATION
RELIEVE STRESS
STIMULATE ACTIVITY
RECALL MEMORIES

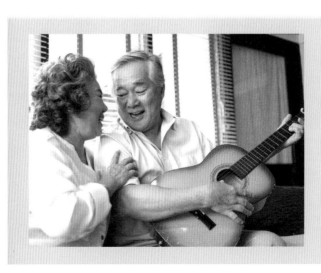
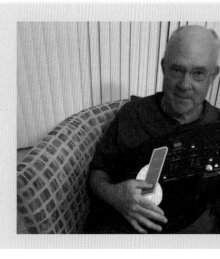

MUSIC! MUSIC! MUSIC!

Music has many benefits for Loved Ones with Alzheimer's. Music can assist Loved Ones with emotional and behavioral challenges. Dr. Jonathan Graff- Radford of the Mayo Clinic has published numerous studies which conclude that "brain areas, linked to musical memory are relatively less affected by the disease".

Music Tips:

- When planning a variety of music observe the Loved One's reaction to determine what music or types of music illicit a positive response. Play music the Loved One likes, and also knows the word

- Be mindful that the volume of played music is extremely important. Played too softly the Loved One may not hear it; played too loudly may result in increased agitation, confusion and stress.

- When you determine what music and volume is enjoyed by the Loved One play it often.

- Music may assist the Loved One during challenging times, such as bathing, by being a calming influence.

- Be mindful that competing noise is most always anxiety provoking. Television in one area, competing with people talking, competing with traffic noise, competing with music in any combination at any time will increase anxiety, stress and discomfort for most of us, but to a greater extent for Loved Ones with the challenges of illness.

- Do not play music that has commercials. Commercials interrupt the Loved One's focus, mood and can be confusing.

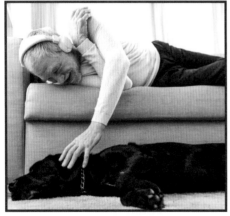 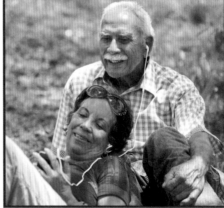 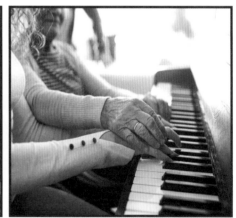

NOTE TO CAREGIVER:

• Be mindful that noted in the "Staged Appropriate" part of this activity it was stated that music is beneficial for most Loved Ones during the early, middle and late stages of the disease. But not all Loved Ones respond in a positive manner to music.

MUSIC ENCOURAGING MOVEMENT

SAFETY PRECAUTION!

✓ Be careful not to overstimulate or create movement beyond the capability of the Loved One. Make it enjoyable and safe. Be specifically mindful of the potential for the Loved One to lose balance, fall or injure themself.

SUPPLIES:

• Music

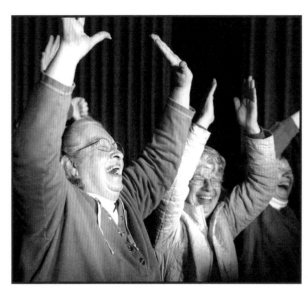

DIRECTIONS:

Caregiver can encourage and direct the following movements:

• Clapping hands
• Tapping feet
• Drumming on a flat surface with fingers and hands
• Chair dancing- while sitting, move arms, legs, and body to the beat of the music. (Be careful that the Loved One is safely seated so as not to fall on the floor).
• Dancing (Be mindful of the Loved One's strength and balance, of tripping and falling hazards and the potential of a Loved One falling).
• Drumming with a safe object on the bottom of an overturned rubber bucket or container.

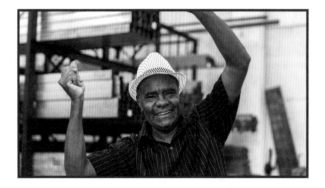

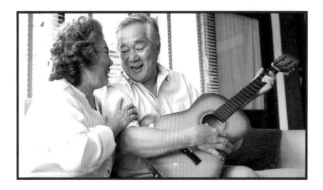

NOTE TO CAREGIVER:

• Please be aware that the selected music or use of percussion instruments may invoke anxiety, stress or fear. Observation and sensitivity to the needs of all present are essential.

Q CHORD MUSIC

Music Fun For All

Easy to learn in a couple of minutes and you cannot make a mistake.

SUPPLIES:

• Q chord Instrument by Suzuki w/plug-in cord
• One or more Suzuki Digital Q Chord Song Cartridges

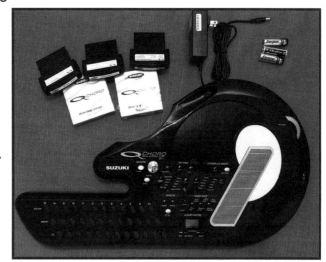

DIRECTIONS:

• It is helpful to watch a demonstration of the Suzuki Q Chord online first.
• Insert batteries.
• Place the Q Cord on a table or hold it like a guitar.
• Insert a song cartridge into the cartridge port.
• Push play button on.
• Run your finger, thumb or hands across the strum plate- any speed, any direction, "any way you want".
• In a few minutes you will be playing "error free" music.

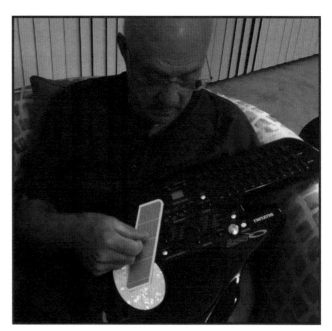

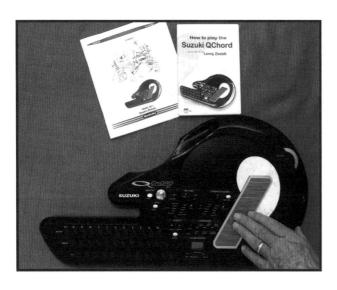

NOTE TO CAREGIVER:

• You, yourself, can enjoy playing this instrument with or without headphones just as much as the Loved One.

SING ALONGS

An Uplifting Activity

The Loved One may well retain the ability to sing along and enjoy this activity longer than you can imagine.

SUPPLIES:

• The voices of the Loved One and caregiver

• A little knowledge of some "old" simple, familiar songs
  Example: God Bless America, America The Beautiful

• DVD'S such as:
  - Sing along with Suzie Q   www.beemusicstudios.com
  - Music for the mind and heart by Katherine Griffin
    www.musicforthemindandheart.com
  - Memory Lane Therapy   memorylanetherapy.com
  - Sing Along For Seniors   melodicmemories.com

• Google or YouTube Songs Examples:
  - Rio's Seniors Sing-along-upbeat
  - Sing Along with Seniors w/printed words
  - Senior Sing Alongs - Dawn Rence
  - Sing Along Elderly Songs
  - What a Friend We Have in Jesus w/lyrics.
  - If you're happy and you know it…
  - 101 Songs (w/lyrics) You Know By Heart
  - John Mc Sweeney

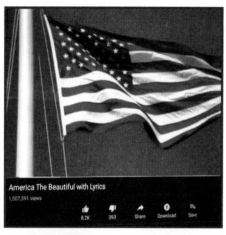

America The Beautiful with Lyrics
1,507,591 views

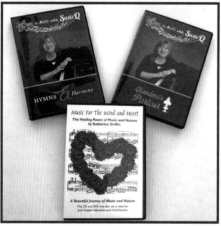

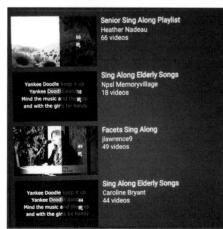

Senior Sing Along Playlist
Heather Nadeau
66 videos

Sing Along Elderly Songs
Npsl Memoryvillage
18 videos

Facets Sing Along
jlawrence9
49 videos

Sing Along Elderly Songs
Caroline Bryant
44 videos

DIRECTIONS:

• Sing loud, sing often, enjoy.

NOTE TO CAREGIVER:

• You can get a plastic bucket, turn it upside down and use a wooden spoon to keep the beat with the music or just tap your foot or hand to the beat.

PAINTING TO MUSIC

Listening, singing, and moving to music activates different parts of the brain, helping to bring up experiences and emotions. Painting does the same thing. Painting to music is even better. It is a nice activity to do together, soothing the soul, and the product , beautiful to look at.

SAFETY PRECAUTION!

✓ Use non-toxic, washable paint, with supervision.

SUPPLIES:

- Favorite soothing music
- Paper
- Paint brush
- Non-toxic, washable paint, variety of colors:
  - blue is very soothing, red, green, yellow are good colors
- Water

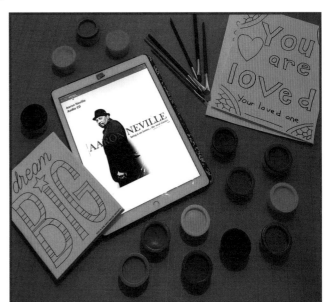

DIRECTIONS:

- Get supplies and music ready.
- Explain that you are going to listen to music and paint along with the music.
- Singing while painting is wonderful as well.
- Caregiver should model the activity, doing it along with the Loved One.
- Talk about what you are painting as well as talk about the music.

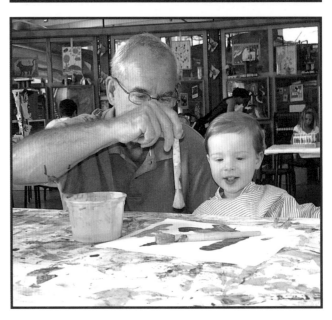

NOTE TO CAREGIVER:

- This activity can be very soothing to the Loved One. Choose a variety of music that you know the Loved One enjoys listening. From this activity, you can go to YouTube, choose a time period, and listen to some favorites. Talk about what you were doing during that time period.

MUSICAL INSTRUMENTS: SHAKERS

This is a fun and free activity to do with the Loved One that will enable him/her to "shake" along with any kind of music.

SAFETY PRECAUTION!

✓ Always be with the Loved One when filling the empty containers. He/she may try putting some of the items into their mouth. After filling the containers, seal well with a glue gun or very sticky tape.

SUPPLIES:

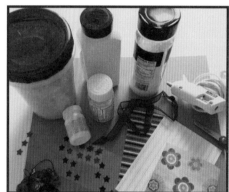

- Empty vitamin/supplement containers (hand held size)
- Empty plastic spice containers
- Colored paper, stickers, markers
- Glue stick, glue gun, tape, scissors
- Dry rice, beans, popcorn kernels, old beads… things that make noise

DIRECTIONS:

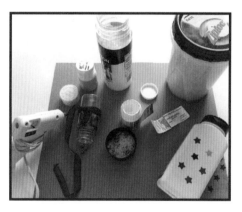

- Remove all items from containers.
- Wash and dry containers.
- Decorate as desired, with colored paper, markers, stickers.
- Fill each one with noisy items, such as dried rice, dried beans, even old beads.
- Secure lid using a hot glue gun or very sticky tape such as duct tape or mailing tape.
- SHAKE, SHAKE, SHAKE to different kinds of music and with different sounding containers!

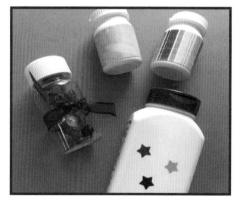

NOTE TO CAREGIVER:

- If you use clear plastic bottles like Bayer Aspirin, the Loved One can see what is inside. Most plastic spice bottles are the perfect size to hold in your hand. Caregiver, you can make one for yourself to use as well!

151

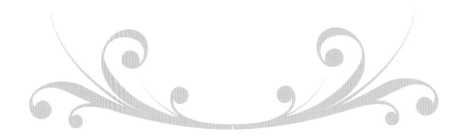

**"Every act of love
is a work of peace"**

– Mother Teresa

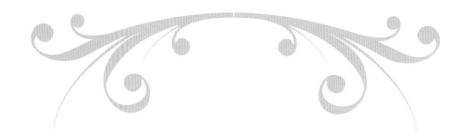

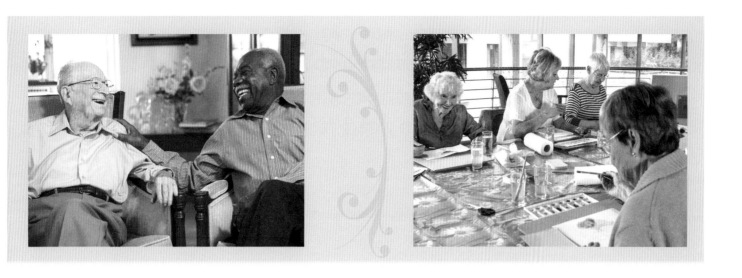

Addendums

A METHOD TO EVALUATE
MEMORY CARE, ASSISTED LIVING
AND NURSING HOME FACILITIES

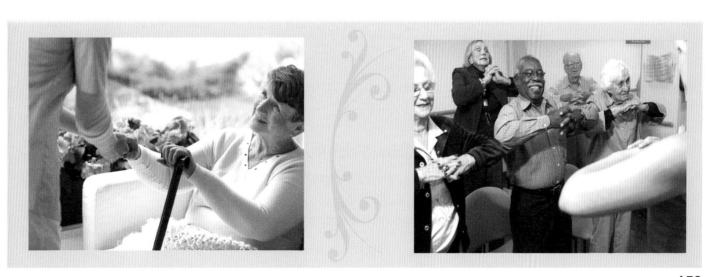

A Method To Evaluate Assisted Living Facilities, Memory Care And Nursing Homes

At some point during the care of your Loved One, there may be a need to utilize the services of outside-the-home facilities.

Various facilities may include: memory care, assisted living, rehabilitation or nursing home care.

In addition to long term care many facilities offer short duration, respite care of a few days or weeks.

The decisions involving utilization of outside services are difficult. Talk to as many people as possible. Consider joining a memory care support group where you can talk with other caregivers who may have had experiences with outside facilities.

If you utilize an outside consultant to identify possible facilities for your Loved One be extremely careful, check out references with other caregivers, and contact a local Alzheimer's Association for information on the consultants services.

Be aware many referral consultants may be employed by or are receiving substantial payments from the facilities they recommend to you and your Loved One.

IMPORTANT!

If you identify a facility for your Loved One, it is strongly recommended you take this one step first prior to entering into any contract or payout a reservation deposit.

Ask if they provide short term respite care services in their facilities. If so use them for a week or so before deciding to enter into a contract or paying out a contract deposit.

This method may be a great way for you and your Loved One to assess services, and determine if a longer term arrangement is beneficial. It may also save you thousands of dollars.

To assist you evaluate facilities there are included in this addendum two checklists. The first checklist is a detailed list with instructions. The second is a short form of the first.

When utilizing a check list make the observations yourself. Spend as much time as you need walking around the facility, talking with various staff members, residents and family members of residents.

Please do not simply give the list to a facility staff member to complete. The answers they give may be only the ones they know you want to hear.

Extended/Long Term Care Facility Check Off (short form)

This form is an alternative to the long form. It is designed to provide a focus on key factors. This form is easier to utilize. However it is recommended that you first review the long form in detail which will provide insight into why the questions are presented in the short form.

A brief overview of State Regulations of Residential Care Facilities and the need to personally evaluate local facilities and services

A person's understanding of what residential care facilities provide for services, or do not provide, can best be understood by reviewing state requirements relative to these type of facilities.

For that purpose one resource is the U.S. Department of Health and Human Services which provides a list of requirements state by state for residential care. The website can be accessed-aspe.hhs.gov.

Following is a very brief overview of some regulations.

Residential care facilities are provided in community based care buildings for individuals who are unable to live at home.

The services and the cost for services vary greatly while basic services that are provided are stipulated and regulated at the state level of government.

Residential care settings generally include:

- Food
- Overnight protection
- Housekeeping
- Laundry
- Transportation
- Social and recreational services
- Staff to assist residents

Each state has some minimal regulations related to nursing care, medication dispensing and staffing when applicable.

A review of nurse staff requirements indicate that they fall into one of three categories:

1. No state requirements for nursing staff
2. A licensed nurse be available through an employment contract or as a consultant
3. A licensed nurse, RN or LPN be on staff

All states have minimal staffing ratios and training for other personal care staff.

Personal care staff is defined as individuals who are <u>unlicensed</u>, but may be required to have some training.

States may have minimal regulations for staff to <u>assist</u> a person take their medications. These staff members are <u>not</u> generally required to be licensed.

Food requirements, except in six states, require three meals per day.

Note: Information on nursing home quality may be found: HHS.gov&medicare.gov

Evaluation Checklist

Memory Care Facilities, Skilled Care Nursing Homes, & Residential Care Facilities

How to use this checklist

This checklist is a FIRST STEP to narrowing down a possible placement for your loved one. Use this checklist - one for each facility - for any level residential skilled nursing care. Some services or programs may not be available in all locations. However all information gathered in response to any of the following questions may be used for comparison purposes between like and similar levels or types of care.

Suggestions

1. Visit at least THREE different facilities owned and operated by DIFFERENT entities.

2. Visit facilities unannounced, three or more times.

a. Make sure at least one visit is on a weekend day, preferably after 3 p.m.

b. Also, visit at different times of day - early morning, noon, late afternoon.

3. Do not judge a program by the appearance of the exterior of the building, which has little to do with the quality of the personal and professional services provided!

A. General Considerations

Question	Yes / No	Comments
What agency licenses and / or accredits the facility?		
Are local state, or federal accrediting agency reports available to review?	Y N	
What criteria are used to evaluate and accept patients?		
Is the facility accepting new patients? If not, what are the waiting list protocols?	Y N	

A. General Considerations (continued)

Question	Yes / No	Comments
What are the facility's discharge policies?		
If for any reason a patient is being discharged, does the patient (or his/her representative) have a right of review and appeal?	Y N	
Is a person's room reserved for his/her return if he/she becomes hospitalized?	Y N	

B. Facilities

Question	Yes / No	Comments
Are there security and fire systems in place?	Y N	
How are community buildings and grounds secured?		
Are there saftety locks on all doors and windows?	Y N	
Are all exits well marked?	Y N	
Are all exits managed in case of an emergency evacuation?		
Does the facility provide various levels of care to address each state of a disease? (If YES, visit each area to see how care differs)	Y N	
Is the facility set up conducive to patient comfort and use...as well as for family and friend visits?	Y N	
Do bathrooms, showers, etc., have grab bars and call buttons?	Y N	
Does the facility have secured outdoor areas for patients and visitors?	Y N	

B. Facilities (continued)

Question	Yes / No	Comments
Does the facility have a lot of common areas for residents' use - lounges, activity areas, walking areas, etc.?	Y N	
Does the facility provide a hospital-type bed, if requested? If so, is there an additional charge?	Y N	

C. Staffing

Question	Yes / No	Comments
* Is the staff visible, friendly, helpful, considerate, and actively involved with residents and visitors?	Y N	
* Are support staff (such as management, nursing director, activities staff, physical therapists, occupational therapists, etc.) readily visible and easily accessible?	Y N	
* How do residents obtain services from physicians (primary care and specialists)?		
How often and when is a physician scheduled to be physically on the premises?		
How are physician services billed?		
* Is an RN on duty in the facility 24 hours a day, 7 days a week? If not, when?	Y N	
* Does the facility conduct background checks on all staff members?	Y N	
* What types of training does the staff receive? How often?		
Is the main entrance staffed at all times when the facility is open to the public?	Y N	

D. Care

Question	Yes / No	Comments
* Does the facility provide for short-term respite care? (This is a great way to evaluate a facility before entering into a contract for extended care.)	Y N	
* Are there any options for a short-term residential trial before entering into a contract for services?	Y N	
* Are ALL residents clean, well-groomed, and dressed appropriately?	Y N	
* What are the protocols and procedures for fall prevention?		
* How often does a resident receive a bath? Where and with what assistance?		
* Does the staff assist residents with eating?	Y N	
Is the food attractive? Does the food taste good?	Y N	
Can you get a copy of the food menu for a month? (Check for variety, choice, appropriateness.)	Y N	
* What are the protocols and procedures for the care of incontinent patients — specifically in reference to the loved one's clothes, bedding, and attention to needs throughout the day and evening?		
Are residents, resident activities, programs, and care grouped by cognitive levels of required care?	Y N	
* Are individual care programs implemented for each resident?	Y N	

D. Care (continued)

Question	Yes / No	Comments
* How often are individual care plans reviewed and changed?		
* Are the family and patient present when individual care programs are changed?	Y N	
* Does the facility have an "aging in place" program?	Y N	
* If so, does the facility provide services for middle-to late-stage care; additional services; and end-of-life care services?	Y N	
Are there any types of care NOT provided?	Y N	
What are the protocols and procedures (physical and medical) for patient restraint?		
What information is available, showing regularly scheduled activities, services, and special programs?		
* Are various therapies offered, including: — light treatment — music therapy — Parkinson's care — pet therapy — physical therapy — recreational therapy — reminiscent therapy — speech therapy — vascular dementia care If so, are there any extra charges for them?	Y N	
* Are resident rights posted?	Y N	

E. Financial

Question	Yes / No	Comments
What are the various room charges?		
What are the extra/optional costs (e.g., medications, incontinence, bath assistance, etc.), and how are they authorized and billed?		
Are there any considerations given that could reduce costs and deposits?	Y N	
Are there charges for prescription medications relative to acquisition and/or administration?	Y N	
Can you obtain a copy of a residential contract to take home and review?	Y N	

1. Day: _____   Time: _____

2. Day: _____   Time: _____

3. Day: _____   Time: _____

4. Day: _____   Time: _____

5. Day: _____   Time: _____

Extended / Long Term Care Facility Evaluation Check Off
(Short Form)

This form is an alternative to the long form. It is designed to provide a focus on key factors. This form is easier to utilize. However it is recommended that you first review The Long Form in detail which will provide insight into why the questions are presented in the short form.

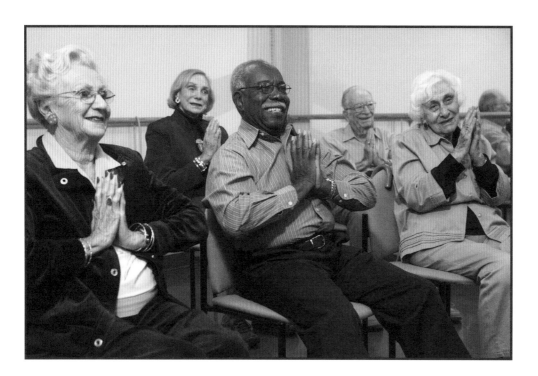

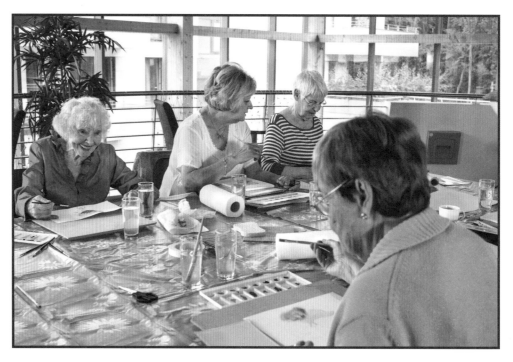

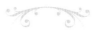

Extended / Long Term Care Facility Evaluation Check Off (Short Form)

Date _____

Observer _____

Name of Facility _____

	Yes	No		Yes	No
Accepts Medicare	☐	☐	Accepts Medicare	☐	☐
Registered Nurse on site 24/7	☐	☐	Licensed Practical Nurse on site 24/7	☐	☐

Admission / Enrollment or Inititaion Fee $ _____   Basic Cost Monthly $ _____

Full Day Care Cost $ _____   Half Day Care Cost $ _____

Respite Care Cost per Day $ _____   Trial Stay Cost per Day $ _____

Additional Fees for Services

_____

_____

_____

	Yes	No	
Does the facility hold beds for Temporary Absence?	☐	☐	If Yes # of Days ____
Are all Areas **CLEAN** and **FRESH** Smelling?	☐	☐	
Are ALL Residents Clean and Well Dressed?	☐	☐	
Is the STAFF Visible and Friendly?	☐	☐	

How and by Whom are Medications Administered? _____

First Impression at Walk-In
10 = Excellent   1 = Poor   ☐

Other

_____

_____